The Beginner's Guide to

LYME
Disease

Diagnosis and Treatment
Made Simple

Nicola McFadzean, N.D.

Foreword by
Joseph J. Burrascano Jr., M.D.

The Beginner's Guide to
LYME
Disease

Diagnosis and Treatment
Made Simple

BioMed Publishing Group

P.O. Box 550531

South Lake Tahoe, CA 96155

www.LymeBook.com

Copyright 2012 by Nicola McFadzean, N.D.

ISBN: 978-0-9882437-1-2

For related books and DVDs, visit us online at www.LymeBook.com.

DISCLAIMER

This book is not intended as medical advice. It is also not intended to prevent, diagnose, treat or cure disease. Instead, the book is intended only to share the unofficial research and opinion of the author. The book is provided for informational and educational purposes only, not as treatment instructions for any disease. Much of the book is a statement of opinion in areas where the facts are controversial or do not exist. The information in this book should not be considered any more valid than any other type of informal opinion.

The book was not written to replace the advice or care of a qualified health care professional. Be sure to check with your own qualified health care provider before beginning any protocols or procedures discussed in this book, or before stopping or altering any diet, lifestyle, or other therapies previously recommended to you by your health care provider. The treatments described in this book may have side effects and carry other known and unknown risks and health hazards.

Lyme disease is a controversial topic and this book should not be seen as the final word regarding Lyme disease medical care. The statements in this book have not been evaluated by the United States FDA. Use of the information in this book is at your own risk.

CONTENTS

ACKNOWLEDGMENTS

FIRST, I WANT TO THANK MY PUBLISHER BRYAN ROSNER FOR HIS motivation, guidance and amazing partnership in this project. Thank you for the time you poured into the manuscript, for the knowledge and experience you brought to it, and the sense of support and camaraderie that you provided for me along the way. Dr. Burrascano, I am deeply honored that you have supported this book—thank you for carving out the time to go through it all; and for your positive feedback and endorsement. It means so much to me.

Thank you to Kim Junker, best friend extraordinaire, for your amazing editing contribution, and also for your friendship and encouragement —we make a great team! To Adriana Covell, thank you for keeping my practice running while I was focused on writing, and for understanding when I wasn't available for other projects. Scott Forsgren and Connie Strasheim, thank you for the time you generously spent on the manuscript and the helpful suggestions you made.

Finally, thank you to all my patients, for allowing me to love the work I do every single day, for the gratitude and appreciation you give me and for allowing me to contribute to you. Your strength and determination to keep moving forward in the face of hardship is inspirational, and it makes me love and respect you all the more.

FOREWORD

I BEGAN MY PRACTICE OF PRIMARY CARE INTERNAL MEDICINE IN 1981 in a small town in coastal New York, known for its natural beauty —untouched pine forests, wetlands, and many wild animals. It is also part of the coastal bird flyway, through which our feathered friends travel as they migrate from one hemisphere to the next. Ominously, it also is located just 30 miles across the water from Lyme, Connecticut.

Soon after I set up my office, in addition to seeing the usual ailments common to this type of medical practice, I did note that there was a surprisingly large population of patients with "strange" illnesses. How could a relatively young person have a degenerated right hip, while the left hip, obviously the same age, was fine? Why so many "atypical" cases of Lupus? And what about the many patients with unexplained brain fog and confusion, to the point of having difficulty making sentences? The nerve "tingles," the insomnia, the fatigue, the head and body aches, the anxiety, the "depression" that always was associated with knee pains?

Well, as I was to find out a few years later, my little town would become noted for having the highest reported case rate of Lyme disease in the world!

Lyme disease is not a new illness. It has been recognized, in one form or another, for over a hundred years. In unraveling its history, one can see many instances of missed opportunities, unrecognized patterns and outright mistakes by scientists, physicians and government officials. Over time, a divide developed between the front-line, Lyme-treating physicians, and the scientists and physicians at our major institutions, both at the university level and in government.

How did this come to be? What have been the consequences? Could any of the troubles we are now facing in the Lyme Wars have been prevented?

My personal Lyme story began in the mid-1980s when the pathologist at my local hospital, the genius Dr. Alan MacDonald, one day invited me to his makeshift "skunkworks," a little lab he created in an abandoned part of the hospital morgue. There he showed me his custom-built microscope, but more importantly he had me look through the eyepiece. And there they were—crazy looking undulating thread-like bacteria that he was able to grow out from the blood of many of my patients. Yes, they were *Borrelia burgdorferi*, the spirochetal bacterium known to cause Lyme disease.

As it turned out, Dr. Willi Burgdorgfer had collected the actual ticks from which he discovered this germ, which was eventually named after him, from a spot within a bike ride from where I lived and worked! He and Dr. MacDonald became friends and colleagues and together they laid the foundation for the modern concept that Lyme disease is in fact an infectious disease.

To gain perspective, one must go back in time a few years. In 1975, after many calls from residents of Lyme, Connecticut, led by Ms. Polly Murray, the U.S. Centers for Disease Control sent Dr. Alan Steere, a rheumatologist and epidemiologist, to Connecticut to study this cluster of unusual rashes and painful swollen joints. Two years later he published a study of 51 cases of a new clinical entity and called it "Lyme Arthritis". He recommended treatment with aspirin and steroids; he considered it self-limited and saw no benefit from treatment with antibiotics. After all, he is a rheumatologist and not an infectious disease specialist.

After the discovery by Dr. Burgdorfer, the need to treat this bacterial infection with antibiotics became accepted. But which antibiotics? At what does? And for how long?

Steere conceptualized Lyme as being an illness that displays both "major manifestations" and "minor manifestations". He and his colleagues defined successful treatment as the elimination of the major symptoms (Bell's palsy, acute carditis, inflammatory arthritis) even though, in Steere's belief, they usually would resolve over time without treatment! They also basically dismissed the minor manifestations—the headaches, fatigue, body pains, confusion, nerve tingles and numbness, etc.

They assumed, without any proof, that the remaining minor symptoms reflected a non-infectious immune-mediated phenomenon, and called it the "post-Lyme syndrome."

Having treated many Lyme patients by then, I recognized that in disseminated disease, ten to fourteen day courses of antibiotics would either result in only a lessening of the illness, or an initial good outcome followed by a relapse. The patients would then respond again to a repeat course of antibiotics. Based on this experience, and looking through Dr. MacDonald's microscope and using his *Borrelia* cultures, it became clear to me that short courses of antibiotics were prone to failure, and that these recurrent or persisting symptoms were due to an ongoing infection. I disagreed with Steere and formulated my own definition of "successful treatment": clearing of all Lyme symptoms, both major and minor, with no relapse by three months after treatment ended.

How does one achieve this? The answer, based on a systematic treatment study I did in 1988, was to increase both the dose of the antibiotics that were then in use, and then to extend the duration of treatment out to several months. The data clearly demonstrated a direct relationship between treatment duration and success. My conclusions, presented at the 1990 International Congress on Lyme Disease in Stockholm:

> "I conclude that each patient responds uniquely and must be managed individually, and more importantly, the duration of anti- biotic therapy is just as important as which antibiotic is chosen in order to achieve a lasting remission."

My work was confirmed independently by many front-line, Lyme-treating physicians from all across America. They included such well known and admired physicians as Drs. John Drulle in New Jersey, Ed Masters in Missouri, and Paul LaVoie in California.

After Steere's original series of articles, the entity known as Lyme Arthritis received official U.S. government recognition. However, instead of assigning the study of this new entity to the infectious disease branch of the National Institutes of Health, immunologists and rheumatologists were given the job. Here began the split between university-based and government-supported researchers (who still claim that persisting symptoms post treatment are autoimmune because they believe, despite evidence to the contrary, that the Lyme infection could not possibly persist after several weeks of antibiotics), and the front-line Lyme-literate physicians who disagree with them.

But what about the patients? Patients with Lyme become torn between front-line Lyme-treating physicians and the University-based clinics. As a result, support groups sprang up all across the United States, and at the same time the first of many non-profit, national organizations formed to advocate for Lyme victims and their families.

Lyme-literate physicians and allied health practitioners eventually joined together to form the International Lyme and Associated Diseases Society (ILADS), a top-level professional organization that has been instrumental in raising the scientific bar, developing meaningful treatment guidelines, and educating physicians worldwide. Finally there is now a blend of hard science with common sense that had been lacking.

Where do we stand now? The Lyme Wars continue, but with a lot of hard work and sacrifice by many, patient and practitioner alike, the truth is getting out there and many more are becoming Lyme-aware. Through this wonderful book and the hard work and in-depth research it reflects, one can now be empowered to proceed on a foundation of knowledge and the security of knowing that you are not alone, that you are not just imagining your symptoms, and that you can be helped. I deeply respect and appreciate this book and hope you enjoy reading it as much as I have. Please accept my best wishes, always!

Sincerely,

Joseph J. Burrascano Jr. M.D. ("Dr. B")

Dr. Burrascano is a well recognized specialist in the diagnosis and treatment of Lyme and associated complex infectious diseases, and the chronic illnesses that accompany them. With over twenty five years of experience and research in this field, he has appeared in and on virtually every form of media both here and abroad, has advised the CDC and NIH, testified before the U.S. Senate, an armed services joint subcommittee, and at various governor's councils.

He is also a founding member of the International Lyme and Associated Diseases Society, and currently is an active Board Member of the affiliated International Lyme and Associated Diseases Educational Foundation.

No longer in clinical practice, Dr. Burrascano works full time in the biotech arena to further medical research in tick-borne and other chronic illnesses.

Notable among many of his ongoing projects is his active involvement in the recent development of in vitro culturing methods of symbiotic Borrelia including the Borrelia responsible for Lyme Disease. This landmark achievement provides a new standard for diagnosing all stages of Lyme disease and can be used to follow the outcome of treatment. Dr. Burrascano is still recruiting practitioners for his ongoing project, "The Lyme and Associated Diseases Registry"™, which follows each selected patient from the beginning to the end of their illness, tracking symptoms, tests, treatments and outcomes. Finally, his lifelong interest in nutrition has come to bear with his present consultative work with various nutritional supplement suppliers.

PREFACE

I STARTED TREATING LYME DISEASE SEVERAL YEARS AGO THROUGH my practice in San Diego, California. I was treating autistic children at the time, and started consulting with some of the children's mothers who were in their 30s and struggling with chronic fatigue and fibromyalgia-type syndromes. It seemed odd to me that so many women were feeling so poorly, but they attributed it to caring for special needs kids and soldiered on. As I worked with them and assessed them for Lyme disease (among other things), I realized how prevalent the illness was, even in California, which is not considered a key region for Lyme disease. Over the next few years, my Lyme disease practice grew and it became my major area of focus.

As part of my work, I have also become involved in the Lyme disease community in Australia, and work with many Lyme patients there, helping them to get an accurate diagnosis and appropriate treatment. At the time of writing the health authorities in Australia still deny the existence of Lyme disease in that country, and so obtaining adequate medical care is extremely difficult for patients. This book, in fact, started out as the basis for a guide to Lyme disease in Australia. However there are many people world wide who are newly diagnosed and desperately need information to help them learn about Lyme disease, and so this next edition is in response to that need.

The connection I have to the Lyme community in Australia has been very rewarding for me, and is natural given that I grew up in Sydney and still consider myself to be Australian. I trained as a naturopath in Australia in the mid-90s but moved to the United States in 1998 and pursued my Doctorate in Naturopathic Medicine, a four-year post graduate program leading to board certification and licensure as a primary care physician in the state of California.

As a licensed doctor in California, I can legally prescribe antibiotics, and I certainly see a place for them in Lyme disease treatment. My training as a naturopath means that I view the body holistically, and see how imperative it is to support the body using natural modalities and nutrition. With most of my patients I use a combination of antibiotic and naturopathic regimens.

My passion comes from seeing a large and ever-growing group of people suffer, and suffer unnecessarily; and out of that comes my commitment to make a difference and a contribution to the world of Lyme disease.

– Nicola McFadzean N.D.

SECTION ONE

SETTING THE
STAGE

1. INTRODUCTION

IF YOU ARE NEWLY DIAGNOSED, HAVE A FAMILY MEMBER WHO HAS been diagnosed, or have recently heard of Lyme disease and are wondering if it might relate to you, chances are, you are experiencing a pretty steep learning curve right now.

On first hearing the words 'Lyme disease,' you might have rushed to look up Lyme on the internet, scanned a few sites, gathered some facts and read some fallacies (the differences between them barely discernible), and sat motionless, stunned, overwhelmed, and devastated. If you are a woman, you may have placed three calls in quick succession to various girlfriends, devoured a box of cookies—the empty container lying on the table next to you—and drank a couple of glasses of your favorite shiraz. If you are a man, you may have decided that your health issues were all in your head, and figured that on the back nine this weekend, it wouldn't look so bad. Unfortunately, as is often the case with the severe nature of this illness, you may already be flat out in bed, unable to do any of these things, wondering what on earth is going to happen next and what it all means for you and your family.

If you are further along the learning curve and already living in the world of chronic Lyme disease, you will know that it can be a complex, confusing, and bewildering place. The complexity of the illness makes navigating its pathways difficult, and the lack of awareness and acceptance of it by the medical community certainly creates massive stumbling blocks.

There is a bright side though—at least now you have a diagnosis, some-thing you can wrap your mind around, a known entity that you can tackle, and a path to pursue towards wellness. Years of misdiagnosis and unending doctor visits with no beneficial results may have left you weary of the whole process, but I encourage you to rally your optimism, appreciate that this is a new road—a road full of new hope and new possibilities—and that even though it may be long and not particularly smooth, it does, at least, provide a renewed path of action and the poten-tial for significant improvement, if not full recovery.

The Purpose of This Book

My hope is that this book will be a tool for you, a resource guide to help you sort through all the information being presented to you so you will feel more empowered to actively participate in your own care. I will share the historical and political context of Lyme, and give a clear description of what Lyme disease actually is, as well as guidance on evaluation and testing, and a wide range of treatment options.

In addition to being written for patients, this book is also written for health practitioners who may be new to Lyme and are trying to get up to speed to help these very sick patients with whom they are consulting, but have not found solutions by following the traditional medical algorithms. Unless they are in the north-eastern regions of the United States, many primary care physicians have not been trained to consider Lyme disease on the list of possible diagnoses, and while that may be frustrating for the many affected people who struggle to find answers and informa-tion, the doctors are not to blame. They are following what the health authorities and medical societies tell them. We need to change that. We need to enhance their knowledge. We need to help them become aware, educated, and willing to address the problem alongside their patients. Clearly we need many more health professionals to be familiar with Lyme disease, so that they recognize it when they see it, and if nothing else, are able to refer out appropriately.

In this book I will also present some of the difficult challenges and complexities of Lyme disease—being realistic while remaining positive about the world of Lyme, and staying aware and therefore armed with knowledge. Knowledge, after all, is power. This illness is disempowering, so now is the time to take a bit of that power back, gather whatever information we have and put it to good use.

I hope to provide a resource that you can refer back to again and again. Please note though, that there is no one course of treatment that will work for everyone; some people may do well on natural treatments while others need hefty doses of antibiotics; some people may improve quite quickly while others may take months or even years. There is no set, clearly defined path that is true for everyone. In trying to present as much practical information as possible, please understand that this book does not substitute for medical advice that is specific to you. The book contains ideas and protocols, not prescriptions.

With that disclaimer in mind, I hope you find it to be a beneficial tool from which you can draw useful information. Many patients have been stumbling alone in the dark, self-diagnosing, self-treating, and propping one another up emotionally, and that takes its toll. It is time to change that, bring this problem into the light, raise awareness and start Lyme sufferers on the road to recovery.

2. THE SCOPE OF THE PROBLEM

ALTHOUGH MANY PEOPLE HAVE NEVER HEARD OF LYME DISEASE, it is actually the fastest growing infectious disease, and the most common vector-borne illness, in the United States.[1]

In 1991, Lyme disease became a "notifiable" disease requiring health authorities to report confirmed cases, and the recorded numbers have risen ever since. In 2000, there were 17,730 confirmed reported cases of Lyme disease. In 2009, that number had nearly doubled to 29,959.[2] The highest reporting rates come from the north-eastern, mid-Atlantic, and north-central states, are among persons aged 5-14 years and 45-54 years, and are highest in the summer. According to the Centers for Disease Control (CDC), there are approximately 20,000 newly reported cases every year.[3]

The statistics above reflect only those cases that have been "counted" according to CDC diagnostic criteria. Who knows what the real numbers are? Who knows how many cases of Lyme disease go undiagnosed and unreported, either because they do not meet the official diagnostic criteria which we will see later are quite narrow and an inaccurate representation of real numbers of Lyme sufferers, or because they are never recognized as being caused by Lyme disease and are misdiagnosed as something else. *The Townsend Letter for Doctors and Patients*, a prestigious and respected periodical, has estimated that the actual number of new Lyme disease cases in the United States may be ten times higher than the numbers the CDC is reporting; that is, closer to 200,000 cases per year!

The CDC itself suggests a similar likelihood.[4] Even with that underestimation, in 2009 Lyme was still the 5th most common nationally notifiable disease. The following table shows the age and gender spread of Lyme disease cases between 2001 and 2010 in the United States.[5] How sad that the highest incidence rates were in males between five and ten years of age! The second highest group is the group that I see the most clinically—men and women between 35 and 55 years of age.

(http://www.cdc.gov/lyme/stats/chartstables/incidencebyagesex.html)

REFERENCES

1. CDC: Centers for Disease Control and Prevention [Internet]. Georgia: Centers for Disease Control and Prevention; Lyme disease data: Fast facts; 2012 Apr 12 [cited 2012 Jun 24]; [about 3 screens]. Available from: http://www.cdc.gov/lyme/stats/index.html

2. CDC: Centers for Disease Control and Prevention [Internet]. Georgia: Centers for Disease Control and Prevention; Lyme disease data: Fast facts; 2012 Apr 12 [cited 2012 Jun 24]; [about 4 screens]. Available from: http://www.cdc.gov/lyme/stats/chartstables/reportedcases_statelocality.html

3. CDC: Centers for Disease Control and Prevention [Internet]. Georgia: Centres for Disease Control and Prevention; MMWR: Lyme disease---United States, 2003—2005; 2007 Jun 15 [cited 2012 Jun 24]; [about 5 screens]. Available from: http://www.cdc.gov/mmwr/preview/mmwrhtml/mm5623a1.htm

4. Roberts DM, Carlyon JA, Theisen M, Marconi RT. The bdr Gene Families of the Lyme Disease and Relapsing Fever Spirochetes: Potential Influence on Biology, Pathogenesis, and Evolution. Emerg Infect Dis [serial on the Internet]. 2000 Apr;6(2) [cited 2012 Jun]. Available from http://wwwnc.cdc.gov/eid/article/6/2/00-0203.htm

5. CDC: Centers for Disease Control and Prevention [Internet]. Georgia: Centers for Disease Control and Prevention; Lyme disease: Confirmed Lyme disease cases by age and sex—United States, 2001-2012; updated 2012 Apr 9 [cited 2012 Jun]; [about 4 screens]. Available from: http://www.cdc.gov/lyme/stats/chartstables/incidencebyagesex.html

3. THE GLOBAL PERSPECTIVE

LYME DISEASE IS ALSO A GLOBAL PROBLEM—IT KNOWS NO international borders, nor borders of race, color, politics, religion or socio-economic status. As people travel and birds and insects migrate, the bacteria are carried far and wide. Strains of Borrelia, the bacteria that causes Lyme disease, have been found in supposedly unaffected areas, and similarly the co-infections of Lyme (again, more on those later) are far-reaching also. And while Lyme disease is recognized in one state or province, a neighboring state or province might authoritatively state, "We don't have Lyme disease here!" Such logic is fallacious and contrary to the way in which Lyme disease moves and spreads across geographic regions.

Global deforestation has broken down the delineation between humans and tick-dense areas. Human expansion has also resulted in the reduction of predators that hunt deer as well as mice, chipmunks and other small rodents—the primary reservoirs for Lyme disease. Researchers are also investigating the role of global warming in the spread of vector-borne diseases such as Lyme disease.

Following is a summary of some of the nations affected by Lyme disease. (Excerpted from Bryan Rosner's *Lyme Disease Annual Report*[1]):

England
The British public has been warned by the Health Protection Agency (HPA) to carefully protect themselves from tick bites due to a "sharp

rise in the number of the blood-sucking parasites and increased cases of Lyme disease in Hampshire, Dorset, and Berkshire." The increase in tick population has been blamed on a "particularly wet and mild summer." According to the HPA, "Lyme disease is a highly infectious disease which is transmitted through tick bites and can lead to blindness, paralysis, and even death if left undiagnosed." Britons are advised to protect themselves by "wearing trousers, using insect repellent and checking their skin for ticks" after visits to the countryside. The HPA also notes that "incidents of Lyme disease have increased by 90% since 2006 across the UK, and New Forest, South Downs, Dorset, and Berkshire have now been named as tick hot-spots."

Sweden and Norway

The Department of Molecular Biology at Umeå University, Umeå, Sweden, released a study in 2007 that stated: "The reported geographical distribution of Lyme disease is constantly increasing in Sweden." The report cites findings, which show that birds play a key role in the spread of Lyme disease due to their long distance dispersal and their role as reservoir hosts for Borrelia. In addition to Lyme disease in Sweden, Swedish researchers also discovered that sea birds in the Arctic region of Norway carry Ixodes uria ticks infected with Lyme disease, specifically the Borrelia garinii strain. It has long been known that Borrelia garinii is one of the more common forms of Lyme disease on the European continent, and this information shows the spread of this strain to new geographical areas.

Russia

In collaboration with U.S. Centers for Disease Control (CDC) researchers, Russian scientists set out to determine which types of bacterial agents are found in the North Western region of Russia. The type of tick examined was Ixodes persulcatus. Researchers discovered the following:

Altogether, 27.7% of ticks were infected with at least one organism, while the DNA of two or more bacteria was found in 11.8% of ticks tested. The highest average prevalence of Anaplasma (20.8%) was detected in ticks from Arkhangel'sk province, while the prevalence in ticks from Novgorod province and St. Petersburg, respectively, was 7.3% and 12.2%. Only

Ehrlichia muris DNA was identified by DNA sequencing. In comparison, the prevalence of B. burgdorferi DNA was 16.6%, 5.8%, and 24.5% in the respective locations.

The Russian researchers conclude with this statement: "Since Ixodes persulcatus is so commonly infected with multiple agents that may cause human diseases, exposure to these ticks poses significant risk to human health in this region."

Germany

Researchers in Germany studied the influence of preventative measures on the risk of being bitten by a tick and suffering from Lyme disease in children attending kindergarten in forested regions of Germany. Fifty-three schools were studied, encompassing 1,707 children. Researchers concluded that "children in forest kindergartens are at a considerable risk of tick bites and Lyme disease."

Poland

Department of Occupational Biohazards investigated the prevalence of Lyme disease bacteria in ticks collected from wooded areas. 1,813 ticks from six districts were examined by polymerase chain reaction (PCR). Not only did researchers discover that a significant portion of the ticks were infected, they also were surprised to find that many ticks were infected with multiple strains of Lyme disease bacteria, including Borrelia afzelii, Borrelia garinii, and a new yet-unnamed strain, "Borrelia b.s.1."

Portugal

A Portuguese University, in a study of climate change, discovered that warmer and increasingly variable weather may result in an increased incidence of vector-borne diseases, including malaria, schistosomiasis, leishmaniasis, Lyme disease, and Mediterranean spotted fever.

Scotland

A fascinating report from the microbiology department at Raigmore Hospital in Scotland states that at least nine different strains of Borrelia have been documented in Scotland, including Borrelia afzelii and Borrelia sensu stricto. Additionally, a report appeared on September 15, 2007, in the *North Scotland Press and Journal,* entitled "Bloodsucking Ticks Blamed as Lethal Lyme Disease Cases Soar." This newspaper article not only documents the dramatic increase of Lyme disease cases in Scotland, it also provides evidence that Lyme disease can be fatal if not treated adequately. The article uses the word "rocketed" to describe the dramatic increase in cases over the past decade. Dr. Ken Oates of Health Protection Scotland observes that "There has been a genuine rise. Nobody can really say why. I would guess a summer like this, which is warm and wet, provides favorable conditions. Up to one in five ticks can carry Lyme disease in Scotland."

Croatia

As far away as Croatia, researchers are finding Lyme disease. Amazingly, 3,317 cases were reported from 1987 to 2003 in Croatia. North-western Croatia showed the highest incidence. According to a report published by the Department of Public Health, "the clinical picture of Lyme Borreliosis in Croatia is dominated by erythema migrans, followed by neurological manifestations."

Switzerland

In Switzerland, according to researchers, "the incidence of tick-borne encephalitis has been clearly increasing since 2004, and this is caused mostly by Lyme disease."

Canada

The Canadian Centre for Disease Control states "the black-legged tick, Ixodes scapularis, has a wide geographical distribution in Ontario, Canada, with a detected range extending at least as far north as the 50th parallel, and four out of five regions of Ontario affected." Additionally, "The Lyme disease spirochete was detected in 12.9% of I. scapularis adult ticks." Also according to Canadian authorities, "characterization of B. burgdorferi in Canada displays a connecting link to common strains of Lyme disease found in the north-eastern United States." According to the Vector-Borne

Disease Laboratory in British Columbia, "In 1994, British Columbia was declared an endemic region for Lyme Borreliosis." In Alberta, Lyme disease has been found to be common in rabbit ticks. The Department of Medicine at McGill University, Montreal, notes in a recent report that "Lyme disease is an expanding community health issue."

The poor recognition of Lyme disease by the medical establishment is not a phenomena limited to the United States: On September 17, 2007, CBS News Canada reported the story of approximately 100 Lyme disease sufferers who gathered on Parliament Hill in Canada to get the attention of Canadian physicians. The aim of the gathering was to get better testing for the disease and more federal money devoted to research—many in the group say they were misdiagnosed by their physicians. Amazingly, according to the CBS report, "Lyme disease is not a nationally reportable disease in Canada, according to the Public Health Agency of Canada (PHAC), meaning there are no statistics available on its prevalence." Yet, although not reportable, CBS goes on to state that "Borrelia burgdorferi is predominantly found in parts of British Columbia, southern and eastern Ontario, south-eastern Manitoba, and parts of Nova Scotia."

Try to figure out that contradiction: not reportable yet found practically everywhere. The CBS article concludes with the story of a Canadian professor who, after suspecting Lyme disease, was forced to travel to the United States and pay more than $15,000 out-of-pocket for treatment. Now, with unrelenting persecution of Lyme doctors in the United States, appropriate Lyme disease treatment may be harder and harder to find... anywhere in the world. The research identifying Lyme disease in Canada goes on and on, with over 83 official, published studies on Lyme disease in Canada. The Canadian Lyme Disease Association can be visited at www.canlyme.org.

Africa

A report published in Africa notes that "Lyme disease is now the most common vector-borne disease in Europe and North America, but there is also evidence that the disease is in Africa as well." Researchers found various strains of Borrelia in ticks located in Tunisia and Morocco, including the strains B. garinii, B. burgdorferi ss, and B. lusitaniae. More than 40 published studies have been released chronicling Lyme disease in Africa. On September 24, 2007, Afriqu' Echos Magazine, one of the larger news magazines in Africa, reported on a team of researchers who, from 1990 to 2003, studied the disease in Dielmo, a Senegalese village. They found that over 11% of Africans in the village had suffered from Borreliosis at one point in their lives. The same article in Afriqu' Echos Magazine also quotes the French Institute of Research and Development (the IRD): "Lyme disease is the most frequent bacterial disease in Africa, but it is also an affliction that is completely unknown to health professionals." The IRD evaluated a rural African area of Dakar and found that "Lyme Borreliosis was the most frequent reason for dispensary consultations after malaria." The article in Afriqu' Echos Magazine further states that:

> "Researchers also discovered that this disease caused recurrent fever in the long term which could result in serious meningoencephalitis, which was sometimes fatal—symptoms exactly similar to those of malaria. The disease is thus systematically confused with malaria, which explains, of course, why there has been so much failure in terms of treatment since treatment for malaria is not effective against Borreliosis. Only tetracycline antibiotics produce results. Diagnosis is also made difficult by the problem of detecting Borrelia crocidurae [note this new strain of Lyme disease], the bacteria responsible for the disease. It is not detectable in the blood except during attacks of fever, and laboratory examinations are rarely possible in tropical Africa, in particular in rural areas."

Imagine the complexity now in Africa of untangling the diagnosis and treatment of two diseases, Lyme disease and malaria, which have similar symptoms and are presently ravaging Africa, but which health care practitioners are not trained to differentiate.

South America
South America is not immune either. Chile, Brazil, Argentina, Costa Rica,

and other countries have reported isolated, although increasing, incidences of the Lyme disease infection. Numerous studies document Lyme disease in South America.

Australia

Case reports of Lyme disease in Australia date back to the early 1980s. Three of them are reported in case reports and letters to the editor in the Medical Journal of Australia. All three meet the diagnostic criteria for Lyme disease. Despite resistance to acknowledge Lyme disease as an emerging disease in Australia, there is increasing evidence of it there. According to the Lyme Disease Association of Australia, at the time of writing there are at least 15,000 diagnosed cases of Lyme disease in Australia, with conservative estimates of another 200,000 people undiagnosed.

A recent study of 51 subjects looked at both Borreliosis and co-infections of Lyme disease in Australian patients.[2] Most patients reported symptom onset in Australia without recent overseas travel. 28 of 51 (55%) tested positive for Lyme disease. Of 41 patients tested for tick-borne co-infections, 13 (32%) were positive for Babesia species and nine (22%) were positive for Bartonella species. Twenty-five patients tested positive for Ehrlichia species and (16%) were positive for Anaplasma phagocytophilum while none were positive for Ehrlichia chaffeensis. Among the 51 patients tested for Lyme disease, 21 (41%) had evidence of more than one tick-borne infection. Positive tests for Borrelia, Babesia duncani, Babesia microti, and Bartonella henselae were demonstrated in an individual who had never left the state of Queensland. Positive testing for these pathogens was found in three others whose movements were restricted to the east coast of Australia. Interestingly, four subjects from this study had not left Australia, and still had positive lab results for Lyme disease and Babesia.

Researchers at the University of Sydney are looking into the diagnostic aspects of Lyme disease in Australia—comparing the results of testing for Borrelia done in Australia, with results of tests run through IGeneX, a specialty Lyme lab. The goal of the research is to assess whether results are comparable from both, and whether the Australian testing is sensitive enough to detect Borrelia; as well as to evaluate whether the U.S. CDC surveillance criteria are appropriate in Australia.[3]

Results so far show that of 148 Australian patients, 70% returned a positive IgG or IgM Western Blot through IGeneX lab in the United States. Further 53% returned confirmation of exposure of up to 3 other tick-borne pathogens (e.g. Rickettsia species, Babesia species, Bartonella species). Put simply, when tested through a specialized lab, with more sensitive diagnostic procedures, 70% of Australian patients showed a positive result while 53% of that group tested positive for co-infections.

■ ■ ■ ■

The above information only scratches the surface. Many more pages would be needed to report all the available studies and articles. It is no great surprise that Lyme disease is emerging as a global epidemic. Geographical borders are simply imaginary lines used to differentiate political systems, allocation of land, leadership organizations, financial infrastructures and other man-made tenets. While some boundaries are physical, in the case of rivers or oceans, there is still migration of birds and animals across borders. Indeed, in many cases borders between countries hold no ecological significance, and thus do not contain microbes or disease processes. So it is with the spread of Lyme disease throughout America and to many nations of the world.

REFERENCES

1. Rosner B, et al. 2008 Lyme disease annual report. South Lake Tahoe (CA): BioMed Publishing Group; 2008 [cited 2012 Apr]. Available from: http://www.lymebook.com/lyme-annual-report.

2. Mayne P. Emerging incidence of Lyme borreliosis, babesiosis, bartonellosis, and granulocytic ehrlichiosis in Australia. Int J Gen Med. Epub 2005 Mar 19.

3. Herzberg G, Hudson B, Mayne P, McFadzean N, McParland B, Mitrovic A, Schloeffel, R. Lyme Borreliosis diagnostics in Australia: limitations, concerns and a way forward. Poster session presented at: The Australasian Society for Infectious Diseases; 2012 Mar; Fremantle, WA; and The Zoonosis meeting at Sydney University; 2012 Jul; Sydney, Aus.

4. A HISTORICAL PERSPECTIVE ON LYME DISEASE

TO UNDERSTAND THE STRUGGLE INHERENT IN THE RECOGNITION, diagnosis and acceptance of Lyme disease, it is important to look at it's history, which is quite fascinating, and may date back further than we think.

It is often cited that the first cases of Lyme disease originated in a specific region in Connecticut in 1975, including the towns of Lyme and Old Lyme. However, descriptions of the illness that is now known as Lyme disease date as far back as 1764. Reverend John Walker was visiting an island off the coast of Scotland, and documented an illness with severe pain in the limbs that he related to a tick vector.[1] Many people from this area of Great Britain immigrated to North America between 1717 and the end of the 18th century, which could have perpetuated the spread between continents.

In the 19th century, the examination of preserved museum specimens found Borrelia DNA in an infected Ixodes ricinus tick from Germany that dated back to 1884, and from an infected mouse from Cape Cod that died in 1894.[2]

Early European studies reflect the skin manifestations of Lyme disease. Swedish dermatologist Arvid Afzelius presented a study at a 1909 research conference about an expanding, ring-like lesion he had observed in an older woman who had been bitten by a sheep tick. He named the lesion *erythema migrans (EM)*, which is now a primary characteristic of Lyme disease.[3]

Neurological problems following tick bites were recognized starting in the 1920s. French physicians Garin and Bujadoux described a farmer with a painful nerve inflammation accompanied by mild meningitis (swelling around the brain) following a tick bite. A large, ring-shaped rash was also noted, although the doctors did not relate it to the other symptoms. In 1930, the Swedish dermatologist Sven Hellerström linked the erythema migrans rash and neurological symptoms following a tick bite.[4]

Incredibly, in 2010, the autopsy of Ötzi the Iceman, a 5,300-year-old mummy discovered in the Italian Alps, revealed the presence of the DNA sequence of *Borrelia burgdorferi*. This fascinating discovery would make him the earliest known human with Lyme disease![5]

The outbreak of Lyme disease in Connecticut in the mid-70s may not have been the first cases of Lyme in the nation, but those cases certainly drew attention to a symptom cluster that did not fit with traditional and well-recognized diagnoses. A group of children in the town of Old Lyme who were affected displayed joint and muscle pain, which may have been in keeping with the diagnosis they were given of juvenile rheumatoid arthritis. However, what linked their symptoms with the possibility of Lyme disease was the presence of neurological symptoms, and the EM rash recognized from European cases.

In 1980, the New York State Health Department provided Willy Burgdorfer, a researcher at the Rocky Mountain Biological Laboratory, with collections of ticks named Ixodes dammini [scapularis] from Shelter Island, NY, a known Lyme-endemic area, as part of an ongoing investigation of Rocky Mountain spotted fever. In examining the ticks for Rickettsia, Burgdorfer noticed spirochetes—spiral-shaped bacteria—in 60% of the ticks. Burgdorfer, familiar with European literature on spirochetes, put two and two together and realized that they might be the cause of Lyme disease. The health department supplied him with more ticks from Shelter Island, and blood samples from patients diagnosed with Lyme disease, and with the assistance of Alan Barbour from the University of Texas Health Sciences Center, he confirmed his discovery by isolating spirochetes identical to those found in ticks from patients with Lyme disease.[6]

In June 1982, he published his findings in the journal *Science*, and the spirochete was named *Borrelia burgdorferi* in his honor.[7]

An intriguing part of the story is the conspiracy theory that Lyme disease was introduced into the north-eastern region of the U.S. by a man-made strain of Borrelia burgdorferi that escaped from a high-security biological warfare laboratory on Plum Island, which sits in Long Island Sound. In 1952, the facility was managed by the U.S. Army Chemical Corps as a component of its biological warfare program. Some claim that the bacteria were "leaked" to the island, made their home in the ticks, which then latched on to the deer, which then swam across Long Island Sound to nearby Connecticut and infected a group of teenagers who were then the first recorded cases of Lyme disease in the United States. The book *Lab 257: The Disturbing Story of the Government's Secret Plum Island Germ Laboratory*[8] by Michael Carroll presents interesting evidence in regards to that view.

While I do not claim to have enough information to be able to sort fact from fiction in this regard, there seems to be ample evidence of the existence of Borrelia burgdorferi long before the 1970s in both the United States and the rest of the world. In fact, in the United States, recent studies revealed that Ixodes ticks and B. burgdorferi were present in the northeastern and mid-western regions in pre-colonial times and many years before European settlements were established in the U.S.

As you can see, many people think Lyme disease is a new, American disease, but clearly evidence supports its existence in various countries dating back a couple of centuries, and perhaps even thousands of years!

REFERENCES

1. Merton N. Lyme disease in the eighteenth century. British Medical Journal. 1995;311:1478.

2. Rymon MM. Disguised as the Devil: How Lyme disease created witches and changed history. USA: Wythe Avenue Press; 2008. 52 p.

3. Afzelius A. Verhandlungen der dermatologischen gesellshaft zu Stockholm [German]. Archives of Dermatology and Syphilis. 1910;101:100–02.

4. Hellerström S. Erythema chronicum migrans Afzelii [German]. Archiv Dermatologie and Venereologie [Stockholm]. 1930;11:315–21.

5. Hall SS. Iceman autopsy: unfrozen. National Geographic. 2011 Nov.

6. Burgdorfer W. Discovery of the Lyme disease spirochete and its relation to tick vectors. Yale J Biol Med. 1984;57(4):515–20.

7. Burgdorfer W, Barbour AG, Hayes SF, Benach JL, Grunwaldt E, Davis JP. Lyme disease: a tick-borne spirochetosis? Science. 1982;216(4552):1317–19.

8. Carroll MC. Lab 257: the disturbing story of the government's secret Plum Island germ laboratory. New York: HarpersCollins; 2004. 289 p.

5. POLITICAL ISSUES IN LYME DISEASE

LYME DISEASE IS FRAUGHT WITH POLITICAL DIVISION AND CON-
troversy, perhaps more so than any other disease. While this largely
stems from within the United States, it unfortunately spills over into
other nations and greatly shapes the recognition and acceptance of
Lyme, as well as the policies and standards of care that are enforced.

CDC Surveillance Criteria

What has become clear is that being "notifiable" and being "accurately
assessed" are two different things. The CDC's surveillance criteria, adopted
in 1994, pose a great problem for the accurate assessment of Lyme disease,
firstly because these criteria are so narrowly defined (for the purpose of
having a high degree of specificity and confidence in the diagnosis); and
secondly, because those criteria were simply never designed to be used for
clinical diagnosis.

Even the CDC acknowledges, "This surveillance case definition was developed for the national reporting of Lyme disease: it is NOT appropriate for
clinical diagnosis." Yet, the definition is repeatedly misused as a standard
of care for healthcare reimbursement, product development, medical
licensing hearings, and other legal cases.

Prior to 1994, Lyme disease was diagnosed based on certain clinical findings along with certain general laboratory findings. The criteria were as
follows:

Clinical Criteria:

1. Erythema migrans rash.

2. At least one late manifestation of musculoskeletal, nervous or cardio-vascular system disorders; and laboratory confirmation.

Laboratory Criteria:

1. Isolation of B. burgdorferi from clinical specimens; *or*

2. Demonstration of diagnostic levels of IgG and IgM antibodies to the spirochete in serum or CSF (could be by ELISA, Western Blot or IFA); *or*

3. Significant changes in IgG and IgM antibody response to B. burgdorferi in paired acute- and convalescent phase samples.

While this criteria did have limitations—mainly that there was a strong emphasis placed on the EM rash which only a small subset of patients actually exhibited—it did have broad enough parameters to catch a wider range of cases, and it had more emphasis on clinical criteria. The lab criteria was *either* the first *or* the second *or* the third option, not necessarily all three.

The new CDC surveillance criteria are more oriented to the detection of early Lyme, and rheumatologic manifestations of Lyme, whereas we know that in reality Lyme has many diverse systemic manifestations, and that the guidelines leave out a host of other symptoms indicative of Lyme. One example is the cognitive dysfunction and neuropsychiatric manifestations associated with Lyme disease. If a patient has a positive Lyme test with symptoms of late neurological Lyme such as memory loss, difficulty concentrating and "brain fog", they would not be diagnosed as a Lyme disease case by the CDC. Why? Because cognitive dysfunction is not part of the CDC's "surveillance criteria" even though they recognize that these symptoms may be attributable to Lyme disease. Their criteria are centered more on the erythema migrans rash, arthritis, Bell's palsy, or early neurological Lyme symptoms involving meningitis or encephalitis (inflammation of the brain and surrounding tissues). The criteria that supposedly aim to achieve accurate assessment and tracking of Lyme disease may actually be preventing many people from getting the diagnosis and treatment they need—and in cases of early Lyme, this may ironically turn a treatable, acute disease into a much more difficult to treat, chronic one.

The CDC surveillance criteria also impact the laboratory testing for Lyme disease by dictating which tests are to be ordered, and what constitutes a positive test result, both to receive a positive diagnosis of Lyme disease, and to meet the criteria to be reportable to health authorities (hence influencing how many cases of Lyme disease are actually recorded).

A two-tiered approach to testing was adopted. The requirement dictated that a positive sensitive ELISA or IFA must be followed by a positive Western Blot with a defined number of approved antibody bands to be considered positive. This created a much more stringent set of criteria, and while those criteria were not intended to be adopted for clinical diagnostics, they were. In particular, they became the standard for insurance companies, for whom a stricter diagnostic criterion means fewer official diagnoses and consequently, less money paid out for patients' medical care.

While the CDC was encouraged to correct the misuse of the surveillance criteria, to date, not much has been done to rectify the problem. Even the passing of Public Law 107-116 in 2002, signed by President Bush, who himself has his own experiences with Lyme disease, has not had a major impact. That law clearly states that the CDC case surveillance definition is unacceptable as a diagnostic tool. Unfortunately it continues to be used and this, combined with the unreliability of laboratory testing for Lyme, has led to misdiagnosis and delayed therapy for many individuals. Yet 99% of practicing physicians are completely unaware of the law and still misuse the surveillance case definition.[1] Part of the necessary education for physicians is to learn the clinical presentations of Lyme disease and make diagnostic decisions based on those, as opposed to following the strict and unrealistic CDC surveillance case definition.

IDSA Treatment Guidelines

Another major barrier to adequate treatment of Lyme disease and a hugely divisive, political phenomenon is the Infectious Disease Society of America (IDSA) stance on acute versus chronic Lyme disease. Where the CDC surveillance criteria are more involved with the diagnosis of Lyme disease, the IDSA guidelines, published in 2006, provide information on the treatment of Lyme disease, including medication dosages and duration of treatment. Those guidelines recognize acute Lyme disease but more or less deny the existence of a chronic Lyme infection, speaking only of "post-Lyme syndrome". According to the IDSA, it is not possible to have the actual infection beyond the acute stage. Any symptoms that exist beyond this stage are just residual symptoms (known as post-Lyme syndrome) that, according to them, are not caused by persistent infection and will resolve by themselves over time.

Not only have these guidelines severely restricted the care available to Lyme patients, they have also been used to prosecute doctors who prescribe outside the limits of their recommendations.

Given the IDSA's thinking that Lyme disease (per their standards) is only an acute and short-term infection, their treatment protocol entails only a short course of antibiotics—between 14 and 21 days. This becomes a significant issue in the world of chronic Lyme disease treatment. If the IDSA publishes guidelines limiting the treatment of Lyme to a maximum of 21 days, then that is what doctors learn and assume to be correct. Furthermore, any doctor who treats outside of those guidelines or standards of care is subjecting him- or herself to scrutiny, censure, and even disciplinary action by the medical boards.

Following are some of the treatment recommendations given by the IDSA, according to the stage of illness:

For early Lyme disease (which by IDSA standards is necessarily associated with erythema migrans "bull's eye" rash, even though in 50% or more of Lyme disease cases this rash never occurs or is not memorable by the patient):

- Simple erythema migrans—doxycycline, amoxicillin or cefuroxime taken orally for 10-21 days.

- For Lyme meningitis and early neurological Lyme disease—ceftri-axone given intravenously for 14 days (up to maximum 21 days).
- For Lyme carditis—oral or parenteral (via intravenous route or intra-muscular injection) antibiotic therapy for 14 days (up to maximum 21 days).

For late Lyme disease (which they do not consider to be "chronic" Lyme disease):

- Lyme arthritis without neurological involvement—doxycycline, amoxicillin or cefuroxime for 28 days.
- Neurological Lyme disease—ceftriaxone via IV for 2-4 weeks.

It is clear that none of the recommendations go beyond a maximum one-month course of antibiotics, with most of them suggesting 14 days only. Yet, according to extensive clinical experience by physicians who have treated thousands of cases of chronic Lyme disease, a four-week course of antibiotics will barely even scratch the surface. Most patients require several months up to a couple of years of treatment to get significant improvements in symptoms. These faulty IDSA recommendations are the key to the disparity between treatment that is needed, and treatment that is being provided.

Furthermore, IDSA guidelines also restrict other treatment approaches that might be attempted, outside of the four or five antibiotics they support.

"Because of a lack of biologic plausibility, lack of efficacy, absence of supporting data, or the potential for harm to the patient, the following are not recommended for treatment of patients with any manifestation of Lyme disease: first-generation cephalosporins, fluoroquinolones, carbapenems, vancomycin, metronidazole, tinidazole, amantadine, ketolides, isoniazid, trimethoprim-sulfamethoxazole, fluconazole, benzathine penicillin G, combinations of antimicrobials, pulsed-dosing (i.e., dosing on some days but not others), long-term antibiotic therapy, anti-Bartonella therapies, hyperbaric oxygen, ozone, fever therapy, intravenous immunoglobulin, cholestyramine, intravenous hydrogen peroxide, specific nutritional supplements, and others." (p.1094)

That's really quite a list of things *not* to do. How can the IDSA possibly verify the "lack of efficacy" for this huge, all-inclusive list of treatments, which even includes "specific nutritional supplements"? It does not seem reasonable that they can categorically dismiss such a range of modalities that have not been individually studied, and yet this broad list was included in their treatment guidelines, which became the medical standard of care.

■ ■ ■ ■

Let us look now at the IDSA view on acute Lyme, post-Lyme syndrome and chronic Lyme disease.

The IDSA talks about post-Lyme syndrome, but there is no recognition of chronic Lyme disease in their treatment guidelines. In fact, they vehemently oppose the possibility of it (page numbers below are in reference to the IDSA guidelines publication, available through their website www.idsociety.org/lyme):

> "There is no convincing biologic evidence for the existence of symptomatic chronic B. burgdorferi infection among patients after receipt of recommended treatment regimens for Lyme disease. Antibiotic therapy has not proven to be useful and is not recommended for patients with chronic (> 6 months) subjective symptoms after recommended treatment regimens for Lyme disease." (p.1094).

So to clarify—the guidelines recognize a continuation of symptoms beyond the treatment regimen, which they term post-Lyme syndrome. They just deny that the symptoms are due to the presence of continued infection in the body.

"The response to treatment of late manifestations may be slow, and weeks to months may be required for improvement or resolution of symptoms after treatment. However, appropriate treatment [their 14 day protocols] leads to recovery in most patients." (p. 1110). They claim that "more indolent forms of neurological Lyme disease are actually quite rare" (p.1110). The reasons given for the persistence of symptoms include ongoing inflammatory processes, residual/irreversible neurological damage or co-infection with other agents such as Babesia (p.1115). At one point, where a tiny window seems to have been opened to the suggestion of persistent infection, somehow those particular microbes seem to be harmless:

> "Even if a few residual B. burgdorferi spirochetes or their DNA debris persist after antibiotic treatment in animal systems, they no longer appear to be capable of causing disease" (p.1119).

My favorites, though, are the implications that ongoing symptomatology is related to the emotional state of the patient, or that the symptoms are in line with what other healthy people experience.

"In many patients, post-treatment symptoms appear to be more related to the aches and pains of daily living rather than to either Lyme disease or a tick-borne co-infection. Put simply, there is a relatively high frequency of the same kinds of symptoms in "healthy" people" (p.1115).

"Previous studies of various infectious diseases have suggested that delayed convalescence can be related to the emotional state of the patient before onset of the illness. In those studies, fatigue was often a persistent symptom. Consistent with these observations, one study of patients with Lyme disease found that poor outcome was associated with prior traumatic psychological events and/or past treatment with psychotropic medications" (p.1116). So ongoing Lyme symptoms correlate with emotional instability prior to the onset of illness? Does this also mean that emotionally unstable people are more likely to attract, and get bitten by, a tick? While I do believe that psycho-emotional elements can contribute to illness, and impact recovery, it is somewhat ridiculous to postulate that the people who are reporting ongoing Lyme symptoms beyond standard 21-day courses of antibiotics are simply manifesting emotional imbalances and prior traumas rather than true infectious processes.

"To summarize, it can be expected that a minority of patients with Lyme disease will be symptomatic following a recommended course of antibiotic treatment as a result of the slow resolution of symptoms over the course of weeks to months or as a result of a variety of other factors, such as the high frequency of identical complaints in the general population" (p.1116). This argument completely fails to acknowledge the thousands of Lyme patients who were completely healthy, or at least asymptomatic, before their tick bite, and now have ongoing and continuous debilitating symptoms despite "appropriate" antibiotic therapy.

Clearly the IDSA is very specific in their diagnostic parameters and treatment protocols and very definite about the acute nature of Borrelia burgdorferi. Their position is happily enforced by medical insurance providers in the United States, who resist covering the costs of long-term medications and care needed for patients.

Of course, the elephant in the room is the thousands of people who have positive lab results for Lyme and/or co-infections and experience health issues following a tick bite; those who have been treated with short courses of antibiotics and still experience symptoms; as well as the thousands who may not necessarily have (for reasons discussed later) positive test results but have the history and symptomatology indicative of chronic Lyme/tick-borne illness.

How can we possibly explain the suffering that is caused by these infectious agents, disabling many, robbing people of quality of life, taking away their feelings of being smart, productive, happy, healthy individuals—saying that the very thing that is becoming a global epidemic does not exist beyond an acute phase, and is "cured" with 14 days of a single antibiotic?

Unfortunately, the misinformation produced by the IDSA guidelines was driven even deeper into traditional medical circles by way of a journal article published in the New England Journal of Medicine (NEJM), one of the most well-respected and credible medical publications in the world.

The article entitled *A Critical Appraisal of "Chronic Lyme Disease"*[2], written by a group of doctors and researchers affiliated with the Infectious Disease Society of America, acknowledges that Lyme disease is the most common tick-borne illness in the Northern Hemisphere, and that it is a serious public health problem. But it's grounding in reality stops there.

The authors recognize that "...after antibiotic treatment, a minority of patients have fatigue, musculoskeletal pain, difficulties with concentration or short-term memory, or all of these symptoms." But, instead of attributing these symptoms to an active bacterial infection, the article states: "Data from controlled trials have shown that there is substantial risk, with little or no benefit, associated with additional antibiotic treatment for patients who have long-standing subjective symptoms after appropriate initial treatment for an episode of Lyme disease." Furthermore, the article dismisses the improvements attained by patients who have received benefit from long-term antibiotic treatment: "Although anecdotal evidence and findings from uncontrolled studies have been used to provide support for long-term treatment of chronic Lyme disease, a response to treatment alone is neither a reliable indicator that the diagnosis is accurate nor proof of an antimicrobial effect of treatment."

Finally, the article concludes by stating that "It is highly unlikely that post–Lyme disease syndrome is a consequence of occult infection of the central nervous system." The following advice is offered to clinicians who see patients claiming to have chronic Lyme disease:

> "How should clinicians handle the referral of symptomatic patients who are purported to have chronic Lyme disease? The scientific evidence against the concept of chronic Lyme disease should be discussed and the patient should be advised about the risks of unnecessary antibiotic therapy. The patient should be thoroughly evaluated for medical conditions that could explain the symptoms. If a diagnosis for which there is a specific treatment cannot be made, the goal should be to provide emotional support and management of pain, fatigue, or other symptoms as required. Explaining that there is no medication, such as an antibiotic, to cure the condition is one of the most difficult aspects of caring for such patients. Nevertheless, failure to do so in clear and empathetic language leaves the patient susceptible to those who would offer unproven and potentially dangerous therapies."

It is not difficult to imagine the damaging and completely counterproductive effects this published article had on sufferers of chronic Lyme disease. This report raised the stakes considerably and rendered an already red-hot, hostile environment, even more perilous.

It is not true and it is not fair, but the big kids in the playground have set the rules, and now hundreds of thousands, or even more, people suffer—through denial of treatment, ridicule, rejection within the medical community, and even rejection by their friends and family members who do not understand the depth and complexity of the illness.

■ ■ ■ ■

Scientific Studies Proving the Existence of Chronic Lyme Disease

In examining the science, it becomes crystal clear that chronic Lyme disease is a true and valid condition. Although much of the research comes from other countries, especially Europe, the following studies show that standard, short courses of antibiotics lead to many treatment failures and relapses, reflecting the chronic nature of the illness.

Some of the following information was excerpted from Bryan Rosner's *Lyme Disease Annual Report.*[3]

Studies Outside the United States

The Institute of Rheumatology, in Prague, Czech Republic reported a case of a female patient suffering from Lyme disease. Her case was confirmed by detection of Borrelia garinii DNA present in her blood and synovial fluid. After treatment with antibiotics, symptoms persisted and six months later, Borrelia garinii DNA was "repeatedly detected in the synovial fluid and the tissue of the patient." Additionally, even after antibiotic therapy, antigens and parts of spirochetes were detected by electron microscopy in the synovial fluid, tissue, and blood.

A similar discovery was made in Germany at the University Hospital of Frankfurt. Researchers described Lyme disease as a "disorder of potentially chronic proportions." They also noted that "therapeutic failures have been reported for almost every suitable antimicrobial agent currently available and resistance to treatment...continues to pose problems for clinicians in the management of patients suffering from chronic Lyme disease."

Another University in Germany, Ludwig-Maximilians-University, located in Munich, reported that "failures in the antibiotic therapy of Lyme disease have repeatedly been demonstrated by post-treatment isolations of the infecting Borreliae."

One of the most interesting German studies, completed at Ludwig-Maximilians-Universitat Munich, attributed the clinical persistence of Lyme disease after antibiotic therapy to the presence of variants and atypical forms of B. burgdorferi. German researchers concluded that "B. burgdorferi produce spheroplast-L-form variants...these forms without cell walls can be a possible reason why Borrelia survive in the organism for a long time."

Researchers at the University of Dermatologische Privatpraxis, Munich, Germany, agreed with their German peers in a 1996 study, which noted that patients with erythema migrans failed to respond to antibiotic therapy. "Persistent or recurrent erythema migrans, major sequelae such as meningitis and arthritis, survival of Borrelia burgdorferi and significant and persistent increase of antibody titers against B. burgdorferi after antibiotic therapy are strong indications of a treatment failure."

In Austria, in 2001, the Lainz Municipal Hospital in Vienna admitted a 64-year-old woman who presented with various systemic symptoms hinting of Lyme disease. When spirochetes were detected in samples of her skin lesions, a diagnosis of Lyme disease was made. According to doctors, "Despite treatment with four courses of intravenous ceftriaxone for up to 20 days, progression of [Lyme symptoms] was only stopped for a maximum of one year."

Researchers at the Turku University Central Hospital, Finland, conducted a study in which 165 patients with disseminated Lyme disease were followed after antibiotic treatment. Approximately 10% of the patients experienced a clinical relapse with positive PCR tests and spirochetes successfully cultured from the blood of the patients. In this case, the Lyme disease relapse was evidenced not only by continuing symptoms, but also by two independent testing methods: both PCR testing and blood culture. This single study, even without aid from the numerous other studies presented in this chapter, should be enough to call into question the IDSA's staunch and dogmatic stance on chronic Lyme disease.

Italy also has experience with chronic Lyme disease. In 1992, the Universita di Genova, located in Genoa, Italy, reported on two patients with "chronic Lyme arthritis resistant to the recommended antibiotic regimens." These patients were eventually cured by long-term treatment with benzathine penicillin. The Italian researchers who conducted this study offered two possible reasons why antibiotic therapy finally worked, and both of these reasons involve active, persistent infection: "The sustained therapeutic levels of penicillin were effective either by the inhibition of germ replication or by lysis of the spirochetes when they were leaving their sanctuaries."

Moving across the globe to Thailand, scientists at KhonKaen University wrote that "Electron microscopy adds further evidence for persistence of spirochetal antigens in the joint in chronic Lyme disease. Locations of spirochetes or spirochetal antigens both intracellulary and extracellulary in deep synovial connective tissue as reported here suggest sites at which spirochetes may elude host immune response and antibiotic treatment."

In France, a study was published in the Journal of Antimicrobial Agents and Chemotherapy in 1996, conducted by the University of Marseille. The study notes that "despite appropriate antibiotic treatment, Lyme disease patients may develop chronic manifestations."

■ ■ ■ ■

Studies Within The United States

It would be understandable for the IDSA to neglect, or at least take less seriously, research conducted outside the borders of the United States, since the IDSA is an organization that operates inside, and is accountable to, U.S. citizens and the U.S. government. However, when we examine studies conducted in the United States, you will see that a significant

portion of the evidence in favor of chronic Lyme disease actually originated on American soil.

In 1996, the Fox Chase Cancer Centre in Philadelphia, Pennsylvania,
conducted a study in which it was discovered that urine samples from 97
patients clinically diagnosed with chronic Lyme disease contained Borrelia burgdorferi DNA. The interesting aspect of this finding is that most
of these patients had previously been treated with extended courses of
antibiotics, the implications of which are simply that antibiotic therapy
(even an extended course) does not always eradicate the infection. The
study concluded that "a sizeable group of patients diagnosed on clinical
grounds as having chronic Lyme disease may still excrete Borrelia DNA,
and may do so in spite of intensive antibiotic treatment."

While the IDSA was releasing their guidelines in which it concluded that
chronic Lyme disease was not a medical condition that justified extended
antibiotic therapy, researchers at the New York State Psychiatric Institute
were discovering just the opposite. The authors of a report produced at
that institution described a case of fatal neuropsychiatric Lyme disease
that was "expressed clinically by progressive frontal lobe dementia and
pathologically by severe subcortical degeneration." Doctors noted that
"antibiotic treatment resulted in transient improvement, but the patient
relapsed after the antibiotics were discontinued...prolonged antibiotic
therapy may be necessary [in some cases]."

In Boston, Massachusetts, researchers at Tufts University School of Medicine conducted a study to investigate neurological abnormalities found
in chronic Lyme disease sufferers; 27 patients were followed. Six months
after a two-week course of intravenous ceftriaxone (2 g daily), 17 patients
showed improvement, 6 had improvement but then relapsed, and 4 had
no change in their condition. Researchers concluded that "months to
years after the initial infection with B. burgdorferi, patients with Lyme
disease may have chronic encephalopathy, polyneuropathy, or less commonly, leukoencephalitis." With regard to the cause of chronic Lyme
disease, Tufts University in their closing statement in the study implies
a bacterial origin: "These chronic neurologic abnormalities usually
improve with antibiotic therapy."

At Thomas Jefferson University, Philadelphia, Pennsylvania, urologists who treated seven patients with Lyme disease found that "neurological and urological symptoms in all patients were slow to resolve and convalescence was protracted...relapses of active Lyme disease and residual neurological deficits were common."

In direct opposition to IDSA statements, researchers at the Department of Pathology, Southampton Hospital, New York, noted that active cases of Lyme disease may show clinical relapse following antibiotic therapy. It is noted that "the latency and relapse phenomena suggest that the Lyme disease spirochete is capable of survival in the host for prolonged periods of time." In their studies of 63 patients with Lyme disease, the researchers concluded that "some patients with Lyme Borreliosis may require more than the currently recommended two to three week course of antibiotic therapy..."

Also in the State of New York, the New York University School of Medicine conducted a study, which evaluated antibiotic treatment of 215 patients between the years 1981 and 1987. Of those with "major" Lyme disease manifestations, a relapse rate of over 20% was observed.

This next study is even more interesting for several reasons, as we will see. The Albert Einstein College of Medicine, New York, reported in 1995 an "unusual" case of Lyme disease in which the patient experienced repeated neurologic relapses despite aggressive antibiotic therapy. What makes this study interesting is that each subsequent course of antibiotics given after the relapses was followed by Jarisch-Herxheimer reactions, which are known to occur only when active bacteria are dying. This implies that active bacteria were still present in the body after multiple courses of antibiotics. Additionally, subsequent to the various courses of antibiotics, the patient's cerebral spinal fluid tested positive "on multiple occasions" for not only complex anti-Borrelia antibodies, but also Borrelia nucleic acids and free antigen proteins. This study demonstrates persistent infection via two separate indicators: repeated Jarisch-Herxheimer reactions, and repeated observation of antibodies and antigens. Both indicators were found after not just one, but multiple courses of "adequate antibiotic therapy" had been administered!

Another similar case observed in Bethesda, Maryland, further calls into question the statement that chronic, persistent Lyme disease infection is "unusual." Doctors in Maryland working with the National Institute of Arthritis and Musculoskeletal and Skin Diseases, a part of the National Institutes of Health (NIH), reported that a 40-year-old Caucasian man who developed clinical Lyme disease after being bitten by a tick was treated with oral tetracycline, after which his symptoms resolved. However, at a later date, the man was re-tested and Borrelia was detected by PCR in his peripheral blood leukocytes. After being re-treated with a longer course of ampicillin, probenecid, and concurrent cytotoxic therapy, symptoms improved significantly. This individual's case of Lyme disease illustrates two important points: First, ongoing symptoms that occurred after antibiotic therapy were confirmed by PCR testing to be caused by active bacteria. Second, re-treatment with antibiotics resulted in significant clinical improvement.

A study published in 2012 demonstrated persistence of Borrelia in monkeys despite antibiotic therapy. Rhesus macaques were infected with B. burgdorferi and a subset of them received aggressive antibiotic therapy four to six months later (antibiotic regimens being doxycycline and/or ceftriaxone). Note that this study was done four to six months post-infection, not immediately, so the infection would have been more disseminated by that point. Subsequent studies via PCR and several other means of testing demonstrated persistence of infection despite antibiotic therapy. This implication of this is recognition that the standard antibiotic protocols suggested by the IDSA are inadequate to eradicate Borreliosis especially once disseminated, and that persistence of infection is possible despite antibiotic therapy.

The other finding of this study is that C6 peptides went down in all treated animals (C6 peptide is an immune marker sometimes used in Lyme disease diagnostics), even though the spirochetes persisted. This demonstrates that chronic infection can be present even with negative antibody tests.[4]

What does the literature tell us? If you take the time to read it and think about its implications, you'll find that the existence of chronic Lyme disease (as caused by an active bacterial infection) is quite obvious and established. Numerous scientific studies conducted across the globe by interdisciplinary scientists have plainly shown this to be the case. The controversy is one of political and dogmatic origin, not of scientific origin. The IDSA denies an active bacterial infection as the cause of chronic Lyme disease not as a result of scientific observation, but instead, because of various inefficiencies and shortcomings inherent in the bureaucratic procedures through which the IDSA operates. The process by which bureaucratic entities accept new truths and grow in knowledge has always been painfully slow and inefficient—and such is the case with the IDSA. Because chronic Lyme disease is in fact real, I am confident that it will be recognized as such sooner or later. Unfortunately, in the meantime, patients are left to dangle in the gap between two sides of an ideological debate.

■ ■ ■ ■

Another falsity that originates from the IDSA guidelines is the limited routes by which Borrelia burgdorferi (and its friends, the co-infections) can be transmitted. The guidelines state that "there is little evidence that a congenital Lyme syndrome occurs" (p.1098) so that rules out mother-to-baby transmission. Also, "unengorged nymphal or adult Ixodes ticks also pose little or no risk of transmission of B. burgdorferi" (p.1098), so that rules out ticks that have been attached less than 36 hours. "Many different tick species bite humans, and some "ticks" removed from humans are actually spiders, scabs, lice, or dirt, and, thus, post no risk of Lyme disease" (p.1099), so that rules out a high likelihood of transmission based on confusion between a tick and a piece of dirt, and also rules out the possibility of transmission by other bugs such as lice or spiders. The guidelines cite the only route of transmission in fact, of any type of Borrelia, is Ixodes species ticks—Ixodes scapularis and Ixodes pacificus. All other ticks are supposedly safe and irrelevant to the conversation. In section two we will examine the evidence that clearly disproves these claims.

The IDSA's slow-turning wheels and "selective filtering of information" are not the only hindrances to its production of accurate and relevant information. In 2006, its entire legitimacy was called into question when an antitrust investigation was launched to investigate its political and ethical motivations.

Former Connecticut Attorney General (now Connecticut State Senator), Richard Blumenthal, announced an antitrust investigation into the IDSA writing of the 2006 Lyme disease guidelines, which are considered the authoritative guidelines on the diagnosis and treatment of Lyme disease. He recognized that the guidelines had sweeping and significant impacts on Lyme disease medical care; that they were commonly applied by insurance companies in restricting coverage for long-term antibiotic treatment or other medical care; and that they strongly influenced physicians' treatment decisions. He also recognized that there were serious flaws in the production of the guidelines:

> "My office uncovered undisclosed financial interests held by several of the most powerful IDSA panelists. The IDSA's guideline panel improperly ignored or minimized consideration of alternative medical opinion and evidence regarding chronic Lyme disease, potentially raising serious questions about whether the recommendations reflected all relevant science."

Blumenthal's findings, as cited on the official State of Connecticut Office of the Attorney General website[5], include the following:

- The IDSA failed to conduct a conflicts of interest review for any of the panelists prior to their appointment to the 2006 Lyme disease guideline panel.

- Subsequent disclosures demonstrate that several of the 2006 Lyme disease panelists had conflicts of interest.

- The IDSA failed to follow its own procedures for appointing the 2006 panel chairman and members, enabling the chairman, who held a bias regarding the existence of chronic Lyme, to handpick a like-minded panel without scrutiny by, or formal approval of, the IDSA's oversight committee.

- The IDSA's 2000 and 2006 Lyme disease panels refused to accept or meaningfully consider information regarding the existence of chronic Lyme disease, once removing a panelist from the 2000 panel who dissented from the group's position on chronic Lyme disease to achieve "consensus."

- The IDSA blocked appointment of scientists and physicians with divergent views on chronic Lyme who sought to serve on the 2006 guidelines panel by informing them that the panel was fully staffed, even though it was later expanded.

- The IDSA portrayed another medical association's Lyme disease guidelines as corroborating its own when it knew that the two panels shared several authors, including the chairmen of both groups, and were working on guidelines at the same time. In allowing its panelists to serve on both groups at the same time, IDSA violated its own conflicts of interest policy.

Blumenthal added, "The IDSA's 2006 Lyme disease guideline panel under-cut its credibility by allowing individuals with financial interests—in drug companies, Lyme disease diagnostic tests, patents and consulting arrangements with insurance companies—to exclude divergent medical evidence and opinion. In today's healthcare system, clinical practice guidelines have tremendous influence on the marketing of medical ser-vices and products, insurance reimbursements and treatment decisions."

It is clear that the very guidelines that drive decisions affecting thousands of people and their day-to-day lives were created by a group that had con-flicts of interest, excluded significant medical opinion that did not support its agenda, and were driven by commercial and financial interests.

■ ■ ■ ■

As much as this kind of ignorance seems like a problem that might relate only to the United States, there is a trickle-down effect that impacts other countries and the opinions of the medical professions there. After all, shouldn't the Infectious Disease Society of America know everything there is to know about an infectious illness like Lyme disease? And shouldn't they be right about it? One would think so; subsequently many doctors look to them for information, read their guidelines, and simply assume that they are accurate and appropriate.

This highlights one of the fundamental issues we face—trying to get chronic Lyme disease recognized in a world where denial by the medical establishment of the very problem that so many people are living with everyday has become the status quo.

On a happier note, the International Lyme and Associated Disease Society (ILADS, www.ilads.org) is a body of clinicians and researchers who have actually studied the science and recognize that chronic Lyme disease is a valid medical problem. ILADS is a non-profit, multinational, interdisciplinary medical society aimed at increasing awareness of tick-borne illness; educating within and outside of the medical community; training physicians and other health care professionals; and sharing guidelines of its own as to testing and treatment protocols for Lyme disease. ILADS is one of the most important resources available for patients and practitioners dealing with chronic Lyme disease, and this organization is growing exponentially as dozens of physicians abandon their old ways of thinking to join ILADS and take their place in the ranks of the growing number of doctors who know how to help people with chronic Lyme disease.

Lyme disease is possibly the greatest medical controversy in history. The political debate between the two sides—the IDSA on one and ILADS on the other, continues. But ILADS is working hard to present the scientific facts of the case—it has published treatment guidelines of its own, and its membership increases every year as more doctors get on board with the reality of chronic Lyme disease.

Interestingly, one of the founding members of the IDSA, Dr. Burton Waisbren, has adapted his stance on the existence of chronic Lyme disease in response to his clinical experience, where he treated many chronically ill patients with Lyme disease. Dr. Waisbren has great influence in the medical community due to his current membership in IDSA and his status as one of its Founding Members. In early 2012, Dr. Waisbren published a book entitled, *Treatment of Chronic Lyme Disease: 51 Case Reports and Essays in Their Regard.*[6] In this book, Dr. Waisbren describes how he now believes that chronic Lyme disease is in fact a real medical condition, and he presents 51 case reports of Lyme disease which he himself has treated, as well as the therapies he used to help these patients. Dr. Waisbren's abandonment of the IDSA Lyme disease treatment guidelines might be seen as a foreshadowing of what is to come, as more and more physicians follow suit in choosing science over entrenched dogma.

Lyme disease has always been controversial, and it has always been misunderstood. I will end this chapter with an excerpt from the book *Bull's-Eye,* on the history of Lyme disease. The author, Dr. Jonathon Edlow, Professor of Medicine at Harvard Medical School, quotes the late Ed Masters, who discovered STARI, a Lyme-like illness:

> Masters points out that the "track record" of the "conventional wisdom" regarding Lyme disease is not very good: "First off, they said it was a new disease, which it wasn't. Then it was thought to be viral, but it isn't. Then it was thought that sero-negativity didn't exist, which it does. They thought it was easily treated by short courses of antibiotics, which sometimes it isn't. Then it was only the Ixodes dammini tick, which we now know is not even a separate valid tick species. If you look throughout the history, almost every time a major dogmatic statement has been made about what we 'know' about this disease, it was subsequently proven wrong or underwent major modifications."[7]

REFERENCES

1. Unknown. Federal Law and a disconnect. In: Lyme MD Blog [Internet]. Montgomery: Montgomery County, MD. 2008 May – [cited 2008 Jun 18]. Available from: http://lymemd.blogspot.com/2008/06/federal-law-and-disconnect.html.

2. Feder Jr HM, Johnson B, O'Connell S, Shapiro ED, Steere AC, Wormser GP; Ad Hoc International Lyme disease Group. A critical appraisal of chronic Lyme disease. N Engl J Med. 2007 Oct 4;357:1422-30.

3. Rosner B, et al. 2008 Lyme disease annual report. South Lake Tahoe (CA): BioMed Publishing Group; 2008 [cited 2012 Apr]. Available from: http://www.lymebook.com/lyme-annual-report.

4. Embers ME, Barthold SW, Borda JT, Bowers L, Doyle L, Hodzic E, Jacobs MB, Hasenkampf NR, Martin DS, Narasimhan S, Phillippi-Falkenstein KM, Purcell JE, Ratterree MS, Philipp MT. Persistence of Borrelia burgdorferi in rhesus macaques following antibiotic treatment of disseminated infection. PLoS One. 2012;7(1):e29914. Epub 2012 Jan 11. Erratum in: PLoS One. 2012;7(4):10.1371/annotation/4cafed66-fb84-4589-a001-131d9c50aea6

5. Blumenthal R. Attorney General's investigation reveals flawed Lyme disease guideline process, IDSA agrees to reassess guidelines, install independent arbiter [Internet]. Hartford (CT): Connecticut Attorney General's Office; 2002 [released 2008 May 1; cited 2012 Jun 5]. Available from: http://www.ct.gov/AG/cwp/view.asp?a=2795&q=414284

6. Waisbren, Burton, Treatment of Chronic Lyme Disease. South Lake Tahoe (CA): BioMed Publishing Group; 2012. Available from: http://www.lymebook.com/

7. Edlow JA. Bull's-Eye: Unraveling the medical mystery of Lyme disease. 2nd rev. ed. New Haven: Yale University Press; 2003. 304 p.

SECTION TWO

FUNDAMENTALS
OF LYME DISEASE

Now that we have looked at the historical and political context of Lyme disease, let us turn to a more thorough discussion of the nuts and bolts of Lyme disease.

6. WHAT IS LYME DISEASE?

BY DEFINITION, LYME DISEASE REFERS TO THE INFECTIOUS ILLNESS caused by the bacteria Borrelia burgdorferi, along with other strains of Borrelia such as afzelii, andersonii and garinii. Borrelia is a spiral-shaped bacterium, known as a spirochete ("spi-ruh-keet"), which crosses over into the blood stream of a human during the bite of an infected tick.

Having said that, the narrow definition of Lyme disease given above, as a strictly bacterial infection caused by Borrelia, may not appropriately reflect the diversity and complexity of the illness. It is more clinically useful to expand the definition to include related co-infections that are transmitted along with Borrelia, such as Babesia, Bartonella, Rickettsia and Ehrlichia. "Tick-borne disease" is another term that may be more inclusive, however, even that limits the recognition of transmission to one vector (the tick), which may not be 100% accurate either.

There are different phases of infection in Lyme disease. Lyme disease is classified according to the longevity of infection, where it has spread in the body and how systemic it has become as well as the types of signs and symptoms it is causing. The earlier the infection can be identified, the greater the success in treatment, which is why awareness of the early forms of Lyme is crucial, including clinical presentations that are not "textbook." It is also important to note that the following phases may not necessarily occur along a linear timeline; some people experience symptoms of advanced, chronic Lyme disease shortly following their infection.

Early Localized Lyme

The classic sign of early local infection with Lyme disease is a circular, outwardly expanding rash called erythema migrans (or EM rash), which may occur at the site of the tick bite three to thirty days after the bite. I say "may" because, in reality, the EM rash is absent in over 50% of Lyme disease cases.[1]

The textbook presentation of the EM rash would be a target shape—a red outer ring with a central clearing—appearing as a bull's eye, hence its nickname "bull's eye rash." Many patients have no recollection of such a rash, or if they think back to a rash they might have had, they may have not recognized it as an EM rash. This is one of the reasons that an acute Lyme infection may not be diagnosed accurately.

The "textbook" presentation of EM rash must also be put in context. One study shows that the tell-tale central clearing was absent in over half of a series of EM rashes examined.[2] Rashes can cover large parts of the body, and they may be patchy or diffuse. They can also mimic other common presentations including a spider bite, ringworm, or cellulitis. In one study, a series of eleven EM rashes were misdiagnosed and treated as cellulitis, with all eleven patients showing clinical evidence of Lyme disease progression.[3]

Along with a rash, early localized Lyme may present with flu-like illness, fevers, malaise, muscle soreness and headache. Lyme disease can progress to later stages even in patients who do not develop a rash. Therefore, Lyme disease should be considered when a flu-like illness is combined with possible exposure through activities such as camping, hiking or gardening.

Early Disseminated Lyme

In early disseminated Lyme, the bacteria spread through the bloodstream and affect other parts of the body. Muscle, joint and tendon pain may appear, often migrating to different parts of the body. Dizziness and headaches, heart palpitations, severe fatigue and mood changes are common.

Neurological symptoms can also start to appear. These include Bell's palsy, which is the loss of muscle tone on one or both sides of the face, as well as meningitis, which involves severe headaches, stiff neck and sensitivity to light. Many people experience burning or shooting pains and unusual skin sensations such as crawling, tingling or burning. Cognitive changes are also common—brain fog, memory loss and difficulty with focus and concentration. Psychological symptoms include severe anxiety, irritability and even the development of obsessive-compulsive traits.

Chronic Lyme Disease

Chronic Lyme disease is trickier to define in light of the Infectious Diseases Society of America's (IDSA) denial of its very existence (see Section 1), but this is the phase of Lyme disease that thousands of people suffer from on an ongoing basis.

Joseph Burrascano, MD, a physician at the forefront of Lyme disease treatment and research in the United States, and author of *Advanced Topics in Lyme Disease: Diagnostic Hints and Treatment Guidelines for Lyme and Other Tick-borne Illness*[4] (a set of treatment guidelines that is widely referenced in the United States, and which is included in an Appendix in this book) offered the following definition:

For a diagnosis of chronic Lyme disease, these three criteria must be present:

1. Illness present for at least one year (this is approximately when immune breakdown attains clinically significant levels).

2. Persistent major neurologic involvement (such as encephalitis/encephalopathy, meningitis, etc.) or active arthritic manifestations (active synovitis).

3. Active infection with B. burgdorferi (Bb), regardless of prior antibiotic therapy (if any).

ILADS, the USA organization that recognizes chronic Lyme disease, has adopted a set of treatment guidelines, which have been widely used in clinical practice (available at www.ilads.org). They state the following:

"Chronic Lyme disease is inclusive of persistent symptomatologies including fatigue; cognitive dysfunction; headaches; sleep disturbance; and other neurologic features such as demyelinating disease, peripheral neuropathy and sometimes motor neuron disease; neuropsychiatric presentations; cardiac presentations including electrical conduction delays and dilated cardiomyopathy; and musculoskeletal problems."

The guidelines also introduce definitions for persistent Lyme disease—symptoms continuing despite 30 days of treatment; recurrent Lyme disease—the patient relapsing in the absence of another tick bite or EM rash; and refractory Lyme disease—a patient responding poorly to antibiotic therapy.

REFERENCES

1. Stricker RB, Lautin A. The Lyme wars: time to listen. Expert Opin Investig Drugs. 2003;12:1609–14.

2. Nadelman RB, Wormser GP. Erythema migrans and early Lyme disease. Am. J. Med. 1995;98(4A):S15–S24.

3. Nowakowski J, McKenna D, Nadelman RB, et al. Failure of treatment with cephalexin for Lyme disease. Arch Fam Med. 2000;9:563–7.

4. Burrascano J. Advanced topics in Lyme disease: diagnostic hints and treatment guidelines for Lyme and other tick-borne illness. 15th. rev. ed. 2005 Sep; Available from: http://www.ilads.org/files/burrascano_0905.pdf

7. HOW IS LYME DISEASE TRANSMITTED?

TRADITIONALLY, LYME DISEASE HAS BEEN CONSIDERED EXCLUSIVELY a tick-borne illness, and while that is no doubt the most common route of transmission, evidence indicates that there are other routes of transmission.

There are a variety of reasons why only 50% of Lyme disease patients recall a tick bite.[1]   First, ticks that most often transmit Lyme disease are in the nymph stage of their lifecycle and are about the size of a poppy seed. Therefore, even in obvious locations on the body, they are incredibly difficult to see or feel. Couple that with the tendency for ticks to gravitate towards less obvious areas of the body such as the scalp, hairline, underarms and groin, and it is easy to understand why identifying them is problematic.

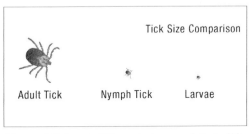

Sizes of ticks at different stages of their life cycle.

Second, ticks numb the skin with an injection of local anesthetic before they actually bite, so that they can remain undetected while attached. This means that people may not feel the bite, or the tick itself.

Third, it is possible that other insects such as fleas, mites, lice and mosquitoes may be able to transmit Borrelia spirochetes to humans and cause infection. Certainly there is clear evidence of those insects housing Borrelia species. Case reports demonstrate illness after bites with mosquitoes and bird mites.

Studies have also shown the presence of Borrelia burgdorferi-like organisms in mosquitoes, horse flies, and deer flies in areas where Lyme disease is present, however, the researchers postulated that those insects were unable to transmit the infections to humans.[2,3]

A Czech study looked for Borrelia and Anaplasma species in chigger mites collected from wild birds. They found through PCR testing that Borrelia as well as the strains of B. garinii, which are known to cause Lyme disease in humans, and B. valaisiana were present in the chiggers.[4]

Also in the Czech Republic, studies proved the presence of Borrelia burgdorferi species in mites from wild rodents, including B. afzelii (also known to cause Lyme disease in humans). Their conclusion was that Borrelia can reside in other vectors besides ticks, and that further study was warranted.[5]

Bartonella, one of the more common co-infections of Lyme disease, has been found in fleas in Australia. The authors described Bartonellosis as "an emerging or re-emerging disease in humans worldwide." In Australia the marsupial hosts included red foxes, bandicoots, rabbits, feral cats, woylies and bush rats. The authors concluded that, "The clustering of Bartonella species with their marsupial flea hosts suggests co-evolution of marsupial hosts, marsupial fleas and Bartonella species in Australia." In simple terms, Bartonella species, which were initially introduced from various hosts following the colonization of Australia, are adapting to Australian animals and the Australian environment to optimize their survival and virulence.[6]

So, the evidence indicates that Borrelia and its co-infections exist in other vectors outside of the tick population, and that further research is needed to evaluate their ability to spread disease.

Is Lyme Disease Sexually Transmitted?

Another major point of contention and controversy is the possibility of the sexual transmission of Lyme disease.

Given that syphilis, also a spirochete bacterium, is sexually transmitted, it seems reasonable to postulate that Lyme may be sexually transmitted also. Outside of simply being spirochetes, both syphilis and Borrelia morph, or transform, into different bacterial forms (including spirochete, cell-wall deficient, and cyst forms) to evade attack by antibiotics and the immune system; they both can remain dormant in their host for years at a time; and they both gravitate to body fluids such as urine, semen, vaginal secretions and breast milk.

There is significant evidence supporting the position that Lyme disease may be sexually transmitted. Dr. Gregory Bach, D.O., O.P.C. from Pennsylvania published an abstract in 2001 that contained telling information from the analysis of his patient population. Dr. Bach had observed that the majority of partners of his Lyme patients were presenting with Lyme disease also, despite only one partner having a history of tick exposure. Further, he noticed that sexually active couples had significantly more antibiotic treatment failures, which led him to believe that one partner might have been re-infecting the other. He continued by analyzing body fluids of his Lyme patients.

He found that:

- Laboratory testing of semen samples provided by male patients (positive by Western Blot and PCR in blood), and the male partners of female Lyme patients, were positive 40% of the time. In the semen itself, Lyme spirochetes were detected in 14 of 32 Lyme patients.

- **ALL** positive semen/ vaginal samples in patients with known sexual partners resulted in positive Lyme titers and/or PCR in their sexual partners.

With evidence of spirochetes found in both semen and vaginal secretions, Dr. Bach rightly concluded that the area of sexual transmission of Lyme is desperately in need of further research.

Of course, the United States CDC (Centers for Disease Control) opposes that view and claims that there is no evidence of sexual transmission at all. They argue that the spirochetes that cause syphilis are structurally and behaviorally very different from those causing Lyme disease, and that basically, they act very differently and do not share the same routes of transmission or pathology. It seems odd that from a genetic perspective Borrelia appears to be a far more advanced pathogen than syphilis, and yet the CDC doubts its ability to be transmitted in bodily fluids.

They also argue that even though it is not uncommon for more than one member of the household to have Lyme disease, the only reason for this could be that they share the same environment so both must have had their own tick bite.

Congenital Transmission of Lyme Disease

Another point of contention is the possibility of congenital transmission— that is, mothers passing Lyme disease to their babies in utero. There is a growing number of children diagnosed with Lyme disease, whose mothers also have Lyme disease and were experiencing symptoms at the time of their pregnancy, even if they were not officially diagnosed at the time.

Once again, while the official government party line is a resounding "No!" to congenital transmission, there certainly seems to be valid evidence.

A study published in the Annals of Internal Medicine reported on a pregnant woman who developed Lyme disease during her first trimester, but did not receive antibiotic therapy. Her infant, born at 35 weeks gestational age, died of congenital heart disease during the first week of life. Histologic examination of autopsy material showed the Lyme disease spirochete in the spleen, kidneys, and bone marrow of the infant.[7]

Another case report described a 24-year-old woman with untreated Lyme disease in the first trimester of pregnancy that gave birth at term to a 2.5 kilogram stillborn. Borrelia burgdorferi was cultured from the liver, and spirochetes were seen in the heart, adrenal glands, liver, brain, and placenta of the baby.[8]

Yet another report was a 37-year-old woman who received penicillin orally for one week for an erythema migrans rash during the first trimester of pregnancy, and subsequently delivered a 3.4 kilogram infant at term who died 23 hours later of what was believed to be "perinatal brain damage." Borrelia burgdorferi was identified in the newborn's brain.[9]

A publication entitled "Maternal Lyme Borreliosis and Fetal Outcome" provided a review of 95 cases of pregnant women with Lyme disease. Antibiotic treatment was administered parenterally—given via injection or intravenously—to 66 women, and orally to 19. Infection remained untreated in 10 pregnancies. Adverse outcomes were seen in 8 of 66 parenterally treated women, 6 of 19 orally treated women, and 6 of 10 untreated women. In comparison to patients treated with antibiotics, untreated women had a significantly higher risk of adverse pregnancy outcome—a full 60% of untreated women had adverse outcomes compared with 12% and 31% of treated mothers (parenteral and oral treatment, respectively). Loss of the pregnancy and cavernous hemangioma (grossly dilated blood vessels and vascular channels) were the most common adverse outcomes.

Further, in this same study when antibiotics were given to the mothers, in 17 cases the EM rashes had not resolved by the end of the course of medication. Adverse pregnancy outcome was more frequent among these mothers than the mothers where the EM rash had resolved.

A study by Alan MacDonald states clearly that transplacental transmission of the spirochete from mother to fetus is possible.[10] He also reports that the variety of manifestations of gestational Lyme Borreliosis mimic the diversity of prenatal syphilis. Among the medical problems are fetal death, hydrocephalus, cardiovascular anomalies, neonatal respiratory distress, hyperbilirubinemia, intrauterine growth retardation, cortical blindness, sudden infant death syndrome and maternal toxemia of pregnancy.

Charles Ray Jones, MD, pediatric Lyme expert, at a presentation given at the ILADS Annual Conference in Toronto, Canada in 2011, stated his opinion that mothers with Lyme disease who were not treated with antibiotics during pregnancy had a 50% chance of passing Lyme on to their baby. In mothers treated with one antibiotic during pregnancy, that likelihood went down to 25%. In mothers treated with two antibiotics during pregnancy, the rate dropped to below 5%.

Research is unclear as to whether Lyme disease can be passed to a baby through breast milk. Certainly, spirochetes, or the DNA of the bacteria, have been detected in breast milk through PCR testing, though the rates and likelihood of transmission through the mother's milk are unknown based on a lack of research data or clinical case studies.[11] Because of this, it would seem prudent to treat a woman who is breastfeeding and has an active Lyme infection with antibiotic therapy, or to advise not to breastfeed, to minimize any risk to the baby.

REFERENCES

1. Steere AC, Broderick TF, Malawista SE. Erythema chronicum migrans and Lyme arthritis: epidemiologic evidence for a tick vector. Am J Epidemiol. 1978;108:312–21.

2. Magnarelli LA, Anderson JF, Barbour. The etiologic agent of Lyme disease in deer flies, horse flies, and mosquitoes. AGJ Infect Dis. 1986 Aug;154(2):355-8.

3. Magnarelli LA, Anderson JF. Ticks and biting insects infected with the etiologic agent of Lyme disease, Borrelia burgdorferi. J Clin Microbiol. 1988 Aug;26(8):1482–86.

4. Literak I, Stekolnikov AA, Sychra O, Dubska L, Taragelova V. Larvae of chigger mites Neotrombicula spp. (Acari: Trombiculidae) exhibited Borrelia but no Anaplasma infections: a field study including birds from the Czech Carpathians as hosts of chiggers. Exp Appl Acarol. 2008 Apr;44(4):307-14. Epub 2008 Apr 10.

5. Netusil J, Zákovská A, Horváth R, Dendis M, Janouskovcová E. Presence of Borrelia burgdorferi sensu lato in mites parasitizing small rodents. Vector Borne Zoonotic Dis. 2005 Fall;5(3):227-32.

6. Kaewmongkol G, Kaewmongkol S, McInnes LM, Burmej H, Bennett MD, Adams PJ, Ryan U, Irwin PJ, Fenwick SG. Genetic characterization of flea-derived Bartonella species from native animals in Australia suggests host-parasite co-evolution. Infect Genet Evol. 2011 Dec;11(8):1868-72. Epub 2011 Aug 12.

7. Schlesinger PA, Duray PH, Burke BA, et al. Maternal-foetal transmission of the Lyme disease spirochete, Borrelia burgdorferi. Ann Intern Med. 1985;103:67-8.

8. MacDonald AB, Benach JL, Burgdorfer W. Stillbirth following maternal Lyme disease. NY State Med J. 1987;87:615-16.

9. (Weber K, Bratzke HJ, Neubert U, et al. Borrelia burgdorferi in a new-born despite oral penicillin for Lyme borreliosis during pregnancy. Pediatr Infect Dis J. 1988 Apr;7(4):286-9.

10. MacDonald AB. Gestational Lyme borreliosis: implications for the fetus. Rheum Dis Clin North Am. 1989 Nov;15(4):657-77.

11. Schmidt BL, Aberer E, Stockenhuber C, Klade H, Breier F, Luger A. Detection of Borrelia burgdorferi DNA by polymerase chain reaction in the urine and breast milk of patients with Lyme borreliosis. Diagn Microbiol Infect Dis. 1995 Mar;21(3):121-8.

8. FACTORS ADDING TO THE COMPLEXITY OF LYME DISEASE

THE NARROW DEFINITION OF LYME DISEASE AS A STRICTLY BACTERIAL illness caused by Borrelia burgdorferi spirochetes is somewhat outdated due to a number of other factors that complicate the issue and must be considered. These complicating factors can create layers of complexity in the realm of chronic Lyme disease.

Complicating Factor #1: Bacterial Strains

There is a great diversity among Borrelia burgdorferi subspecies—over 100 strains in the United States and 300 strains worldwide. In the game of life called "survival of the fittest," the ability of a microbe to adapt, morph, create new strains and create strains that act differently is crucial to its ability to evade the immune system, avoid any therapy that might kill it, and prosper in its ecological surroundings. That ability allows the microbe to establish a permanent domain, not just a temporary home, creating the chronicity of illness we see in Lyme disease.

Some of the strain variations of Borrelia that have been identified in various continents include:

North America: B. burgdorferi, B. americana, B. andersonii, B. bissettii, B. californiensis, B. carolinensis, B. garinii, B. kurtenbachii and B. lonestari

Canada: B. burgdorferi, B. bissettii

Europe: B. burgdorferi, B. afzelii, B. bavariensis, B. bissettii, B. garinii, B.

finlandensis, B. lusitaniae, B. spielmanii and B. valaisiana

<u>Asia</u>: B. afzelii, B. garinii, B. lusitaniae, B. sinica, B. valaisiana and B. yangtze

<u>Japan</u>: B. garinii, B. japonica, B. tanukii, B. turdi and B. valaisiana

All of these strains have been isolated from ticks and animals, but not all have been proven to cause disease in humans. The three strains most recognized to cause Lyme disease are B. burgdorferi, B. afzelii and B. garinii. B. lonestari is also reportable to the CDC in the United States as Lyme disease.

Amongst Borrelia there are currently 14 known genospecies. This diversity of strains is significant because each strain may act differently. For example, the Borrelia burgdorferi, which is responsible for much of the Lyme disease in the U.S., presents differently than B. afzelii and B. garinii, which are more common in Europe. The European strains appear clinically with more neurological symptoms than B. burgdorferi.

Bacteria adapt genetically to fit their environment. It is survival of the fittest, even at that microscopic level. Variations occur over time and in different ecosystems, giving the microbe more and more resilience. This creates a more complex situation for humans to research, study and adapt to in ways that are clinically beneficial for the person suffering from the disease.

Complicating Factor #2: Bacterial Forms

The Borrelia bacterium is a sneaky and wily bug, and it can actually morph into three distinct forms—again, with the view to evading the immune system and gaining a stronger foothold in the body. The three forms are the spirochete, the cell-wall deficient form, and the cyst form.

In very simple terms, think of them as a caterpillar, a cocoon, and a butterfly, respectively. These are three different manifestations of the same creature, according to the position in their life cycle. In each phase, the creature looks very different and acts very differently—some phases are more vulnerable to attack by outside forces than others, some are more resilient. Some impact the environment around them more than others. So, too, the three different forms of Borrelia bacteria look and act differently from the other forms, and impact their environment differently. One of the fundamental distinctions here, however, is that the butterfly cannot really decide he wants to revert back to a caterpillar when it suits him, whereas a Lyme spirochete can go from one form to another in a non-linear fashion. A Lyme spirochete, when threatened, can morph into a cyst form, or become cell-wall deficient. It is a survival mechanism for the bacteria, but one that makes it all the more complex for us to understand and treat effectively.

These three forms are so important to us clinically because all three must be addressed for treatment success to occur, and each form has wildly different susceptibilities to the available therapeutic options.

The form of Borrelia that we hear about most is the spirochete form, or the spiral-shaped form of the bacteria. It is most often implicated in early, acute Borrelia infections. Even in chronic infection, the spirochete forms cause more of the conventionally recognized symptoms, such as flu-like illness, Bell's palsy, and the bull's eye rash. Since the spirochetes are spiral-shaped bacteria, they penetrate the tissues easily, drilling their way into tissue and bone. Their mobility contributes to the multi-systemic characteristics of Lyme disease—the spirochetes do not contain themselves to any one organ or system within the body.

The cell-wall deficient form is the form that may cause the most problems in persistent, chronic illness. They can be hard to treat, as the lack of a cell wall makes targeting by antibiotics and the immune system difficult. They can trigger autoimmune disease, and can be responsible for the numerous syndromes and conditions not typically associated with Lyme disease, such as paralysis, multiple sclerosis, psychiatric manifestations, and chronic fatigue syndrome. The cell-wall deficient forms clump together in colonies deep within the body and can be very challenging to treat effectively.

Often, antibiotic therapy is given to address a single form of the bacteria, which actually can cause more trouble down the road. If only the spirochete or cell-wall deficient form is treated, the bacteria may respond by morphing into a different, more defensive, cystic form. Spirochetes tend to do that when they feel threatened or are under attack. With the spirochete load reduced, the patient may feel better for a period of time, especially since cystic forms do not necessarily cause symptoms, but in this scenario, the bugs are not gone, they are just in hiding. As soon as treatment stops, the cyst forms can return to spirochete forms and the patient is back to square one. However, the patient may be in a worse situation because now, their body has been compromised by the side effects of significant antibiotic therapy. Combining different antibiotics and therapies that inhibit cyst form development is the key to a successful recovery. This will be discussed in detail in section three. Finally, to make matters even more complicated, it has been shown that a single spirochete which has converted to cyst form may re-emerge from cyst form later only to have multiplied into five spirochetes; so the bacteria can actually reproduce while at the same time undergoing transformation from one form to another.

With the three forms of Borrelia—the spirochete, the cell-wall deficient form, and the cyst form—we have a triple-layered problem, and we need a triple-layered solution. Fortunately, different classes of antibiotics have different activity according to the varying structures and traits of bacteria, so there are ways to combine them to address all three forms. This requires prescribing doctors to layer different medications, a minimum of three at a time (or two consistently plus one pulsed), and for physicians who are less familiar with the workings of the wily, Lyme bacteria, this may seem like an overly aggressive approach. I hope with a greater understanding of the various forms of the bacteria outlined in this book, and with the detailed treatment suggestions for each form, physicians will see how crucial this approach is to effectively treating chronic Lyme disease.

Complicating Factor #3 – Co-infections

Co-infections have already been mentioned and will be discussed in light of symptoms, testing and treatment later in the book. What is important here is to understand how prevalent co-infections are, and how they add complexity to the Lyme disease picture.

In that picture, we see several key co-infections, which operate along-side the Borrelia. They are Bartonella, Babesia, Ehrlichia and Rickettsia. With the exception of Babesia, which is a parasite, the other microbes are bacteria.

One point to distinguish here for the purposes of this book is "co-infections of Lyme," versus "opportunistic infections that we commonly see in Lyme disease." For example, Mycoplasma species and Chlamydia pneumonia are other infections that we commonly see in Lyme patients. Epstein-Barr, Cytomegalovirus and Human Herpes Virus 6 are chronic viruses that many Lyme patients carry. Candida albicans, which is naturally occurring yeast in the gut, is often overgrown in Lyme patients (independent of antibiotic therapy). However, I will not refer to them as co-infections because they are not necessarily transmitted along with the Borrelia via an infected tick; rather they are opportunistic and are often present in Lyme patients because of the immune suppression and increased susceptibility of Lyme sufferers. Bartonella, Babesia, Rickettsia and Ehrlichia can be transmitted in the same tick bite as Borrelia, and so that is why I refer to them in this book as the co-infections of Lyme.

According to Richard Horowitz, MD, who has treated thousands of Lyme cases, when he started treating Lyme disease 20 years ago in New York, he believed that most of his patients were simple Lyme patients (without co-infections). Today, he states that over 80% of his patients carry at least one co-infection, with many having multiple co-infections.

One of the challenges of co-infections is identification. As with Lyme disease, diagnosis of co-infections must primarily be based on the clinical picture—that is, a patient's signs and symptoms. Reliable lab testing for most co-infections is challenging—there are many false negatives, and results are not always definitive.

The second challenge is that the co-infections require different treatment protocols than the actual Borrelia infection. Bartonella, Ehrlichia and Rickettsia are closer in structure to Borrelia, since all of them are bacteria. Babesia, however, is an intracellular parasite. Therefore the antibiotics that work for Borrelia are not going to adequately address Babesia. Treatment durations and dosing schedules may also differ for co-infections.

It is possible to weave treatment protocols together to work on a number of different infections at once, but it requires an understanding of different medications and their interactions to create a safe and effective protocol. Many doctors feel hesitant to prescribe multiple antibiotics to cover the different forms of Borrelia as well as the co-infections that are present, but this is often necessary for recovery to occur. Sometimes a combination of antibiotics and herbal antimicrobials can be used to address co-infections concurrently.

In my opinion, missing a co-infection in diagnosis, and/ or under treating co-infections, is one of the biggest factors in Lyme disease treatment failure. Many co-infections go undiagnosed, and while addressing Borreliosis will lead to improvement, that improvement is limited without also recognizing and treating the co-infections. In fact, many Lyme disease researchers now hypothesize that some of these co-infections act to protect Borrelia, such that Borrelia treatment may be ineffective or minimally effective unless co-infection treatment is also successfully administered.

Complicating Factor #4 – Biofilm

Technically, biofilm is a polysaccharide matrix that can be produced by colonies of bacteria such as Borrelia. In simple terms, biofilm is sticky goo that the bacteria produce and subsequently hide in. There are many different types of biofilm. For example, plaque production in the mouth is the result of biofilm from oral bacteria, and there are biofilms in the gut also. Some biofilms serve a beneficial purpose in the body—not all are detrimental—however, several types of infectious microbes produce biofilm around themselves. It is postulated that up to 80% of infections involve some kind of biofilm, and this can complicate the treatment process.

Just as humans form communities to prosper and ensure survival, bacteria do also. The biofilm they create clumps them together, anchors them to tissues and gives them a protective film. This can make them harder to target by the immune system, and it gives them a shield against antibiotics and other antimicrobials. Alan MacDonald, one of the pioneers in biofilm and Lyme disease investigation, discovered that the DNA of the bacteria actually constituted part of the biofilm matrix. Elements such as calcium, magnesium and iron are also present. All forms of Borrelia (cyst, L-forms and spiral forms) have been found within biofilms.[1]

Eva Sapi, PhD, a researcher from the University of New Haven, has also been at the forefront of research on biofilms and Lyme disease. Her research showed that certain enzymes such as nattokinase and lumbrokinase are effective in breaking down the biofilm matrix. The herbs samento and banderol were also effective. This has possible implications for treatment regimens for chronic Lyme disease, and will be discussed in more detail later.

■ ■ ■ ■

It is clear that Lyme disease is not a straightforward health problem; rather it is complex and complicated. Therefore, it is important to be aware of all the different elements of Lyme disease so that it can be treated adequately. There are many other complicating factors involved in Lyme disease, such as parasitic infections, heavy metal toxicity, nutrient deficiencies, chronic inflammation, hormone dysregulation, and others. Some of these will be covered later in this book; others can be researched in other books and resources.

REFERENCES

1. MacDonald AB. Summation of Biofilms of Borrelia burgdorferi. Biofilms of Borrelia burgdorferi and clinical implications for chronic Borreliosis. Lyme Disease Symposium; 2008 May 17; New Haven, CT; p. 71. Available at: http://www.molecularalzheimer.org/files/Biofilm_New_Haven_ppt_Read-Only_.pdf

9. SIGNS AND SYMPTOMS OF LYME DISEASE

Lyme Disease, The Great Imitator

Lyme disease is known as the "Great Imitator." Its list of symptoms is long and varied, and it can present differently in different individuals. A child with a diagnosis of autism may be showing the neurological manifestations of Lyme disease while an individual with a diagnosis of osteo- or rheumatoid arthritis may be showing more musculoskeletal manifestations.

Following is a list of illnesses that Lyme disease can mimic:

- Amyotrophic Lateral Sclerosis (ALS)
- Attention Deficit Disorder
- Autism
- Chronic Fatigue Syndrome
- Crohn's Disease
- Encephalitis
- Fibromyalgia
- Interstitial Cystitis
- Irritable Bowel Syndrome
- Juvenile Arthritis
- Lupus
- Meningitis
- Motor Neuron Disease
- Multiple Sclerosis
- Obsessive-Compulsive Disorder

- Parkinson's Disease
- Psychiatric Disorders (depression, bipolar, OCD etc.)
- Raynaud's Syndrome
- Rheumatoid Arthritis
- Scleroderma
- Sjogren's Syndrome
- Thyroid Disorders

And that is just a sampling.

Lyme disease can trigger autoimmunity, so some people will present with rheumatoid arthritis, lupus, Sjogren's, Hashimoto's thyroiditis or any number of autoimmune diseases. It may not be that these diagnoses are incorrect; it may just be that the Lyme infection has unbalanced the immune system sufficiently to trigger the autoimmune mechanism. Where there is autoimmune disease with sufficient evidence of Lyme disease (either through lab work or clinically), treating the Lyme will often improve, if not eliminate, the autoimmunity.

The key concept to grasp here is that of underlying cause. Western medicine has somehow distanced itself from the quest for discovery of the underlying cause of illness. As is the case with fibromyalgia or chronic fatigue syndrome, the diagnosis describes a set of symptoms but does not explain why they occur. Granted, often chronic fatigue syndrome is preceded by an acute viral illness, but even patients without the acute phase will be given the diagnosis of chronic fatigue simply based on, you guessed it, their symptom of chronic fatigue. Because Western medicine only looks at symptoms, many disease pictures with varying symptoms may be thought to be different diseases because they have different symptoms, when in fact the underlying cause may be singular: Lyme disease.

Clues to Lyme disease being causative are:

1. An individual has a constellation of symptoms involving multiple body systems.

2. Traditional diagnostic tests do not lead to anything conclusive or any clear diagnosis. ("Your tests came back normal. There's nothing wrong with you.")

3. An official diagnosis can be made (such as one of the above) but standard medical treatment does not have the expected benefit or result.

4. A therapeutic trial of anti-Lyme treatment (such as a course of antibiotics) leads to Herxheimer reactions and subsequent symptom improvement.

Since Lyme disease shows such a great variety of symptoms in every possible body system, it does not always fit any classic disease picture. Here is a fairly comprehensive list of the possible symptoms of Lyme disease (reproduced with permission from the Canadian Lyme Disease Foundation, www.canlyme.org):

Skin

- Rash at the site of the bite
- Rash on other parts of the body
- Raised rash, disappearing and recurring
- Striae (stretch marks) that may be red or purple
- Scratches on the skin (like cat scratches)
- Lumps (nodules) under the skin

Head, Face, Neck

- Unexplained hair loss
- Headaches, mild or severe
- Seizures
- Pressure in head, white matter lesions in brain (MRI)
- Twitching of facial or other muscles
- Facial paralysis (Bell's palsy)
- Tingling of the nose, tongue, or cheek
- Facial flushing
- Stiff or painful neck
- Jaw pain or stiffness
- Dental problems (unexplained), tooth pain
- Sore throat, clearing throat a lot, phlegm, hoarseness, runny nose
- Difficulty swallowing, feeling as if something is stuck in the throat

Eyes/Vision

- Double or blurry vision
- Increased floaters
- Pain in the eyes, or swelling around the eyes
- Hypersensitivity to light
- Flashing lights
- Phantom images in the periphery of vision

Ears/Hearing

- Decreased hearing in one or both ears, plugged ears
- Buzzing in the ears
- Pain in the ears, oversensitivity to sounds
- Ringing in one or both ears

Digestive and Excretory Systems

- Diarrhea
- Constipation
- Irritable bladder (trouble starting, stopping)
- Interstitial cystitis
- Upset stomach (nausea or pain)
- GERD (gastro esophageal reflux disease)

Musculoskeletal System

- Bone pain, joint pain or swelling, carpal tunnel syndrome
- Stiffness of joints, back, neck, tennis elbow
- Muscle pain or cramps
- Fibromyalgia
- Tendonitis

Respiratory and Circulatory Systems

- Shortness of breath
- Air hunger - cannot get full/satisfying breath
- Chronic cough
- Chest pain or rib soreness
- Night sweats or unexplained chills
- Heart palpitations or extra beats
- Endocarditis

- Heart blockage

Neurological System

- Tremors or unexplained shaking
- Burning or stabbing sensations in the body
- Weakness, peripheral neuropathy or partial paralysis
- Pressure in the head
- Numbness in the body, tingling, pinpricks
- Poor balance, dizziness, difficulty walking
- Increased motion sickness
- Light-headedness, wooziness

Psychological/ Psychiatric

- Mood swings, irritability, bipolar disorder
- Unusual depression
- Disorientation (getting or feeling lost)
- Feeling as if you are losing your mind
- Over-emotional reactions, crying easily
- Too much sleep, or insomnia
- Difficulty falling or staying asleep
- Narcolepsy, sleep apnoea
- Panic attacks, anxiety
- Obsessive-compulsive traits

Cognitive

- Memory loss (short or long term)
- Confusion, difficulty in thinking
- Difficulty with concentration or reading
- Speech difficulty (slurred or slow)
- Word finding difficulty
- Stammering speech
- Forgetting how to perform simple tasks

Reproduction and Sexuality

- Loss of sex drive
- Sexual dysfunction
- Unexplained menstrual pain, irregularity

- Unexplained breast pain, discharge
- Testicular or pelvic pain
- Vulvodynia

General Well-being

- Phantom smells
- Unexplained weight gain or loss
- Extreme fatigue
- Swollen glands/lymph nodes
- Unexplained fevers (high or low grade)
- Continual infections (sinus, kidney, eye, etc.)
- Symptoms seem to change, come and go
- Pain migrates (moves) to different body parts
- Early on, experienced a "flu-like" illness, from which you have not recovered completely
- Low body temperature
- Allergies/ chemical sensitivities
- Increased effect from alcohol and possibly more intense hangovers

That is quite an impressive list for such a tiny bacteria, but it is a true representation of what Lyme sufferers experience. If asked to check the boxes on a list, many Lyme patients would have 30 or 40 of the above checked.

What makes it all the more devastating for Lyme sufferers is that often-times they do not appear as sick as they really are. Certainly, on the inside, they feel like death warmed over, but outwardly they do not have any major observable manifestations. In fact, I often hear stories of their closest family members, co-workers and friends saying, "But you look so good. Surely you're not that sick?" It is another reason why doctors miss the gravity of their situation; their outward presentation does not always match their inward experience.

■ ■ ■ ■

Can You Guess the Disease?

Given what you now know about Lyme can you tell which disease is being described?

#1 Who Am I?

I could potentially put you in a wheelchair. When I produce some numbness and tingling, you'll probably go and see a neurologist. They will do an MRI and tell you that you have white lesions on your brain, but they will also tell you that there is not too much you can do about it. Or, they may find nothing, and suggest you see a counselor for hypochondria, so you may spend years thinking you are crazy and have no real health problems.

#2 Who Am I?

I make you really, really tired. I mean really tired. It's easy to think of me as something that lingers after a more acute illness. I make it so that you just can't bounce back. The fatigue is overwhelming, and your doctors tell you that you are just doing too much. They suggest that perhaps you need a vacation, or to slow down at work. You know it's more than that, but your blood work doesn't show any real problems and I make it look like nothing is really wrong with you. Mostly you're just tired and wondering if you'll ever get your spark back.

#3 Who Am I?

Within a few months, I can take you from a healthy, happy individual, to one completely unable to care for yourself. I sap your muscle strength and ability to move. I'll impact your legs and arms, and you will require help to move around. Later, when you are lying in bed, you'll need help lifting your arms and being fed. I might seriously impact your ability to eat, and even breathe. Ultimately, I may take your life.

#4 Who Am I?

I give you headaches, and I make you tired. You are grumpy and irritable all the time. I give you night sweats. Your other female friends go through similar things, but somehow this seems different. I work in cycles so every four weeks it seems worse, but I'm also making you sick at other times too, so it doesn't quite make sense. You see your ob-gyn and she checks your hormones, and they may be off so she gives you prescription hormones. You take them but I don't go away.

#5 Who Am I?

I make you hurt all over. Your muscles just ache and it's hard to get any relief. You are really tired, too, and proper and refreshing sleep seems to be elusive. I make you feel sick and tired, but it looks as if there's nothing wrong with you. Your doctors tell you that you're depressed and want to put you on anti-depressant medication. It helps a bit so you think that you might be on the right track, but then you start forgetting things and words are harder to put together. You wonder if it's because of the medications so you stop them, but nothing changes. Every day you wake up exhausted no matter how many hours you've slept.

#6 Who Am I?

I make your joints very sore and stiff. They are swollen, they are hot to touch, and they are red. I take the fun out of life because I stop you from being able to move around too much. Certainly sports and fitness are out of the question. I trick you because you feel well enough to be active, but your joints just won't allow it. You go to the doctor and he does some labs and says, "Yes, you have an illness." Then he tells you the treatment is steroids to combat the inflammation. He doesn't know you have an infection and that immune suppression will make you worse in the long run. In desperation you say yes and it helps then, but over time, things get worse. You gain 20 kilos out of nowhere, and sink into depression.

#7 Who Am I?

You have a small child, and you think your world is just perfect, but you notice your child is not hitting his milestones. Development seems delayed. It's your first child so you don't think too much of it, but then you realize that it's not quite right. You take your little guy to the pediatrician who assesses him and says that there is indeed a problem, although from that point he doesn't seem to have too many ideas for solutions. You go home devastated, thinking that this is just something you will have to live with and adapt to the best you can.

■ ■ ■ ■

Here is what these cases have been diagnosed (and possibly misdiagnosed) as:

1. Multiple sclerosis.

2. Chronic fatigue syndrome.

3. Motor neuron disease.

4. Female hormone imbalance.

5. Fibromyalgia.

6. Rheumatoid arthritis.

7. Autistic-spectrum disorder.

So how did you do? Did you recognize the above descriptions as some commonly diagnosed diseases and syndromes? What appears to be one disease may actually be Lyme disease in disguise, and so in the abovementioned cases, the patients' recovery was jeopardized by a faulty diagnosis.

Symptoms of Co-infections

We have already established that in many cases Lyme disease actually involves a range of different microbes (called "co-infections") such as Borrelia, Bartonella, Babesia, Ehrlichia and Rickettsia. While there is significant overlap between the symptoms of each one, there are also a few clues that can help determine which co-infections are present in an individual. Given that so much of the Lyme diagnosis is based on a clinical picture, health practitioners should understand the co-infections and their hallmark symptoms in order to determine which treatments will best help their patient.

Borrelia

- Gradual onset of symptoms
- Multi-system – e.g. joint pain along with cardiac involvement; cognitive deficits with fatigue and muscle/ joint pain
- Migratory pain from joint to joint
- Fatigue and lethargy, worse in the afternoon
- Four-week cycles
- Stiff, crackly joints
- Headaches originating in the neck
- Slow response to treatment with initial flare (Herxheimer reaction), improvement over weeks with monthly symptom flare
- EM rash in 25% to 50%

Bartonella

- Gradual onset of initial illness
- Central nervous system symptoms out of proportion to musculo-skeletal
- CNS irritability including muscle twitches, tremors, insomnia, seizures, agitation
- Anxiety, severe mood swings, outbursts and antisocial behavior; OCD traits
- Headaches – feel like ice picks in the head
- Gastritis or abdominal pain, bowel problems (IBS)
- Tender sub-cutaneous nodules along the extremities, especially the outer thigh, shins, and triceps
- Occasional lymphadenopathy (swollen, enlarged lymph nodes)
- Striae or stretch marks that are new, out of place, can be white or red/ purple in color
- Pain in the sides and back of the ribs
- Pain in soles of the feet, painful to walk in the morning
- Tachycardia (rapid heart beat)
- Photophobia (light sensitivity)
- Rapid response to treatment but a rapid return of symptoms if treatment is stopped too early

Babesia

- Night sweats and sometimes day sweats as well
- Shortness of breath, air hunger, sighing
- Dry, chronic cough
- Fullness in the throat, difficulty swallowing
- Severe headaches - dull, all over head, feels like head is in a vice
- Dizziness, light-headedness
- Capillary angiomas especially on breasts
- Vasculitis (red skin with white splotches)
- Hormone imbalance
- Easy bruising
- Burning symptoms
- Head/ tooth/ sinus/ jaw symptoms
- Bell's palsy
- Nausea
- Ear ringing
- Blurry vision
- Vivid/ violent dreams, nightmares
- Flushing
- Flare-ups every 4-6 days
- Failure to respond to Lyme treatment
- Feeling of spaciness, wooziness, and impending doom

Ehrlichia/ Anaplasma

- Rapid onset of initial illness
- Headaches – sharp, knife-like, and often behind the eyes
- Muscle pain, not joint pain, can be mild or severe
- Neurological symptoms – seizure disorders, shooting pains
- Tendon pain
- Pain in the right upper quadrant of the abdomen
- Low WBC count, elevated liver enzymes
- Rapid response to treatment

Rickettsia

- Fever/ chills
- Headaches

- Confusion
- Aching muscles
- Gastrointestinal symptoms – nausea, loss of appetite
- Swelling of lymph nodes
- Malaise

10. TESTING FOR LYME DISEASE

TESTING FOR LYME DISEASE IS YET ANOTHER ASPECT THAT FUELS THE controversy and exacerbates the issue of misdiagnosis and under-diagnosis of Lyme. This is because many Lyme tests are not sensitive enough to catch all cases. This is truer of some types of tests than others, as we will see.

The thing to stress before we launch into a discussion on lab testing for Lyme disease is that Lyme disease is primarily a clinical diagnosis which can be made based on a person's history, symptom picture and physical examination. Laboratory findings should be used to back up, or confirm, clinical presentation. Many cases of Lyme disease are not diagnosed because of negative lab results, even in the face of a textbook presentation of signs and symptoms, or a strong enough case history to warrant the diagnosis. In many cases a therapeutic trial of an agent that would kill the Lyme bacteria, such as an antibiotic or an herbal antimicrobial, can give valuable clues into the presence of infection. Theoretically, if the person did not have Lyme disease, a course of antibiotics would not dramatically affect their symptom picture. An antibiotic trial that validates the Lyme diagnosis might give a response of either an improvement, or a worsening of symptoms consistent with a Herxheimer reaction (this will be explained in more detail in later sections). Either way, some shift in symptoms would be expected.

In Section One in our discussion of the inherent political challenges in Lyme disease, we learned that the CDC surveillance criteria were initially designed for epidemiological purposes, such as to track prevalence of Lyme disease cases. They were never meant to be used for diagnostic purposes.

As a reminder the CDC surveillance criteria entail a two-tiered approach to testing, and dictate that a positive sensitive ELISA or IFA must be followed by a positive Western Blot with a defined number of approved antibody bands to be considered positive.

We will see, however, that this two-tiered approach is a flawed system and leaves many people inaccurately diagnosed, and without the medical support and treatment they need.

■ ■ ■ ■

So that you know what all these tests are, let us get some definitions and descriptions out of the way.

In broad terms, tests for Lyme disease can be categorized as direct and indirect.

- Direct tests look for the bugs or parts of the bugs in various body tissues and fluids. Direct tests include PCR, FISH, cultures and biopsies, and antigen-capture tests.
- Indirect tests measure a person's immune reaction to the bugs. Indirect tests include ELISA, IFA and Western Blots for Borrelia, and IgG and IgM antibody tests for co-infections.

Lab testing efficacy is determined by sensitivity and specificity. Sensitivity is how likely the test is to find the infection if it is present. A highly sensitive test has a high probability of finding, or measuring, a particular criterion. Specificity, on the other hand, is how accurate a test is in measuring a particular organism, species, or substance. If a test is specific it will clearly define a marker, without too much variability, confusion, false positives or false negatives. In other words, a highly sensitive test will find a needle in a haystack. A highly specific test will tell you for sure that it is a needle.

Direct Tests

PCR

PCR stands for Polymerase Chain Reaction. It is a test whereby the DNA, or genetic material of the bacteria, is detected in the blood, serum or other bodily fluids such as the cerebrospinal fluid (CSF) or urine. The downside of the PCR test is that the bacteria often like to hide in the tissues, not simply float around in the blood, so they are difficult to detect. The upside is that the PCR test is not dependent on immune reactions or immune function. A person with a dampened immune response is just as likely to show a positive PCR as a person with a strong immune response. This may not be true of indirect tests, which rely heavily on immune response.

A PCR test that detects a spirochete in the blood is quite specific. While there is some possibility of a false positive, a spirochete visualized is a spirochete visualized; it is specific. The test is not that sensitive, however, as spirochetes may not be easily found in the blood due to their burrowing and hiding in the tissues. If the spirochetes are not hanging out in the blood stream, looking for them there may be a futile endeavor. For this reason PCR tests may be more useful in the early stages of infection when spirochetes are more likely to be in the blood.

PCR testing is also limited by the number of Borrelia strains it can identify. Since there are several strains of Borrelia worldwide known to cause disease in humans, a PCR must assess a range of those strains to be most sensitive.

Culture

The culture test for Borrelia has not been widely used clinically to date, although a culture test is now available in the United States.

In a culture test, a small amount of the patient's blood is removed from their body and introduced into a specific medium that promotes growth of a certain type of bacteria. The bacteria that grow are identified by their cell characteristics and growth characteristics, further confirmed by immuno-staining. To go one step further, PCR testing can be run and various strains identified from the sample. In simple terms, the blood sample is put into a specific medium, allowing some time for the Borrelia to grow, then double-checked that it is Borrelia by examination of its traits and its DNA.

The Borrelia culture is a step forward in that it is deemed more reliable than the Western Blot test, and more sensitive than a PCR. Advanced Laboratory Services, Inc. in Pennsylvania, USA, now offer a spirochete/ Borrelia culture test, which at the time of writing it is only available within the United States.

Advanced Laboratory Services, Inc.
501 Elmwood Ave
Sharon Hill PA 19079
855-238-4949 (ph)
855-238-4946 (fax)
www.advanced-lab.com

Biopsy

A biopsy is another direct test as it measures the actual microbes, not an immune response to a microbe.

Biopsies are tissue samples that are taken from almost anywhere on the body and evaluated for different infections. Although biopsies are not commonly done in the Lyme community, they can be helpful especially when there is a localized zone of infection, such as at the site of a recurring EM rash. Biopsies are also sometimes done to assess small fiber nerve degeneration, which is linked with neuropathy and progression of Lyme disease.

A biopsy is a more invasive procedure than a blood draw, and is not among the first-line lab tests performed to evaluate or diagnose Lyme disease.

Lyme Direct Antigen Test

An antigen capture test looks for Borrelia bacteria, or parts of Borrelia bacteria, in the urine. Again, it is a direct test as it is not relying on an immune response but rather looking for the microbe itself. The antigens are parts of the Borrelia bacteria—when isolated from the urine, they are combined with rabbit antibodies specifically targeted to B. burgdorferi antigens. These antigen-antibody complexes are treated with a color developing solution, which turns blue-purple and shows the presence of the Borrelia.

The urine antigen test is often done with a "provocation." By giving antibiotics a few days prior to the collection, thus provoking the bacteria, we can accelerate their destruction making their remnants more likely to show up when measured in the urine.

Indirect Tests

ELISA test

The ELISA test, the problem child of Lyme testing and diagnostics, is the mostly widely run test in the general medical community, and also one of the least useful. Unfortunately, it is the test that is used as a first port of call for many doctors, and a negative result on the ELISA, also used as a screening test for Lyme disease, is used, often incorrectly to rule it out. The ELISA test is offered by many labs worldwide and is often covered by insurance (in fact, insurance often requires that it be the first test run, and will not cover other tests without the ELISA).

There are some fundamental problems with relying on the ELISA test to diagnose Lyme disease. First, the ELISA test does not have adequate sensitivity to fit the two-tiered approach recommended by the CDC. The group responsible for Lyme disease proficiency testing for the College of American Pathologists stated that a screening test must have at least 95% sensitivity to provide an adequate screen, and that the ELISA test simply does not have that level of sensitivity.[1]

In fact, studies have shown that in patients with culture-positive Lyme disease, only 65-70% show an antibody response. Therefore, a full 30-35% of confirmed Lyme cases would have been missed with ELISA testing alone.

To understand how indirect tests such as the ELISA work, we must understand some basic facts about the immune system.

Antibodies are immune cells, and there are two different kinds of antibodies that are evaluated in Lyme testing (and really, testing for any infection). One is the IgM antibody and the other is the IgG antibody. Typically an IgM antibody is going to present much earlier in infection, approximately two to four weeks after exposure. The IgM antibody may stay elevated, indicating an ongoing active exposure. It may also convert to an IgG response. The IgG antibody has a slightly different role. It is not a "first responder" like the IgM antibody. It comes in later, after several weeks of infection, and may stay elevated for long periods of time—months or even years after the initial infection.

Think of the IgM antibodies as the marines (M for marine). They are the first on the scene when there is a threat or invasion; they attack first and ask questions later. The IgG are the ground forces (G for ground). They let the marines check out the situation first then come into play later, maybe several weeks or even months later. Both arms of this immune system military are necessary and have their strategic roles. The timing of each becomes relevant according to which diagnostic tests are ordered in which time frame post-infection.

Even though they are first on the scene, even the IgM antibodies take a few weeks to appear, typically within 2-4 of the initial infection. One can see then, that a patient presenting with an EM rash a few days after infection needs to be immediately evaluated and diagnosed clinically. By the time antibodies appear, the infection may already have been present for a few weeks and valuable treatment time been lost. I would go so far as to say that a flu-like illness with a known exposure to ticks, such as through camping or hiking, should be viewed this way.

IgG antibodies can be confusing as they can also show exposure to an infection without an active infection. An example of this might be after a vaccine, where a variant of a microbe is introduced to the immune system to force it to have an immune response. That way, IgG memory cells are formed, and if that individual encounters the infection again, the IgG memory cells recognize it right away, direct the immune system into action (quick, send in the Marines!) and mount a quicker, more efficient response to the microbe. IgG antibodies may reflect an individual being exposed to Borrelia without becoming sick with it.

One of the problems with this testing is when it measures immune response. Since Lyme disease is known for dampening (weakening) the immune response, this becomes very problematic. The bugs in this case reduce a person's capability to mount an immune response—the indirect tests such as ELISA are measuring an immune reaction—and so negatives arise even in the presence of disease. Further, in more chronic infections, IgG antibodies may be absent 50% of the time, posing further complications for diagnosis in chronic illness.[2,3,4] Subsequently we also evaluate IgM antibody response in persistent or recurrent disease.

The other limitation of antibody testing is that if an individual is treated with antibiotics early, to the extent that the infection is mostly eradicated, it can reduce or completely quell their antibody response. Therefore, they could test negative but still have some infectious process in their body. At a later stage, if symptoms return, most of the antibody markers may not be present.

ELISA testing is also hampered by the actual testing methodology. Testing must be developed to detect more unique and specific antigens for Borrelia. Most commercially available kits use a whole cell sample of the Borrelia microbe. More sensitive testing would recognize and use smaller, more specific pieces of the bug that are known to be reactive, not the whole thing lumped into one.

We can see a double-pronged problem with the ELISA testing. First, the test itself is not sensitive enough. Second, the Borrelia microbe curtails immune response so that the signals necessary to trigger a positive result are lower. Together, it is a profoundly unreliable system.

Let's use the analogy of sound. If a microphone recorded sound, it would need the sound to be at a certain decibel (volume) level to be able to record it, but the microphone would also need to be of good quality with a decent level of sensitivity. If either the volume was too low or the microphone was of low quality (not designed to record lower and higher notes, just the central ranges), then the sound would not register or be accurately recorded. If both were present—poor sound output *and* low microphone quality—the chances of a great recording would be doubly jeopardized.

This is how it is with ELISA testing for Lyme disease, and why it is so crucial to combine laboratory findings with the clinical picture to make an accurate diagnosis. Indirect lab tests alone, especially ELISA tests, leave a lot to be desired in terms of sensitivity, and many very ill patients will go undiagnosed. Despite CDC guidelines and their two-tiered approach, a negative ELISA test cannot rule out Lyme disease and should never be used as a stand-alone test.

IFA Test

Another indirect test is the Immuno Fluorescence Assay, or IFA test. It detects antibodies against B. burgdorferi, but it pools the various antibodies (IgG, IgM and IgA). Therefore, it is looking for an immune response but is not as variable based on time after infection *in comparison with* the ELISA. The IFA is typically run in conjunction with Western Blots. It should not be used *instead of* a Western Blot.

The IFA test is useful when run with other tests, to make up part of the picture. It is not necessarily a stand-alone test and is not necessarily diagnostic in and of itself. While concerns have arisen over time as to the specificity of the IFA for Lyme-specific antibodies and for its potential for cross-reactivity with antibodies to other spirochetes, studies have shown that with high quality testing procedures and highly experienced lab technicians, the IFA test has good specificity and sensitivity. Therefore the IFA should be run through a lab that specializes in Lyme testing to increase its validity.

Western Blot Test

The Western Blot test is one of the foremost tests used in the evaluation of Lyme disease. It is also an indirect test, as are the ELISA and IFA;

however it is a more sensitive test if performed by a laboratory that looks for all the bands that are related to Borrelia. IgM and IgG antibodies are evaluated separately, with the IgM being detected as early as one week post-exposure.

Unfortunately, as has been the case with anything so far relating to CDC criteria, the CDC has also played a role in creating limitations in Western Blot testing and reporting.

A Western Blot reports certain numbers, or "bands," which can be positive, negative, or indeterminate. The bands represent certain antigens, which are the parts of the bacteria that the immune system reacts to.

There is a discrepancy as to which bands are clinically significant, and how many of the bands need to be positive to get a positive result. FDA-approved, commercially available kits (such as the Mardx Marblot) are restricted from reporting all of the bands. These rules were set up in accordance with the CDC surveillance criteria. Private laboratories that are not beholden to these rules and criteria are free to produce tests that actually help people get an accurate assessment.

In IgM testing, by CDC criteria, two of the following bands must be positive to record a positive result:

23-25 kDa
39 kDa
41 kDa

IGeneX, on the other hand, a U.S. based specialty Lyme lab, recognizes the following bands as clinically significant and relevant to Lyme disease:

23-25 kDa
31 kDa
34 kDa
39 kDa
41 kDa
83-93 kDa

Their research has shown that the 31, 34 and 83-93 bands are significant and quite specific to Borrelia infection. The 41 band, on the other hand, shows a lot of cross-reactivity with other flagella-bearing organisms, so a positive 41 can be indicative of other types of infections.

Clearly, the expanded IGeneX criteria give a more rounded and inclusive view of Lyme immune recognition, and allow for a more clinically helpful assessment. Many Lyme-literate medical doctors and experts in Lyme disease believe that just one positive or even equivocal of the above bands is clinically significant.

The other benefit of IGeneX testing is that the bands are reported according to a range—from IND (indeterminate, or weak positive), +, ++, +++ all the way through to ++++. The stronger the immune response to a band, the more +'s are reported. Therefore, even if a patient's test results are negative, but they have, for example, two IND bands (an IND does not "count" as a positive band), it gives clues that the person may be affected by Borrelia. It may seem logical that the more +'s a patient has, the more aggressive and severe their infection, but in fact the opposite might be true. Because Lyme disease disables the immune system, sometimes the sickest individuals have a lower immune response and a 'less positive' looking test result; it does not mean they are any less sick.

The IgG Western Blot has even more stringent criteria than the IgM Western Blot. At least five bands must be positive (out of a possible 10) to be regarded as positive according to the CDC. The test looks for 10 bands: 18, 23-25, 28, 30, 39, 41, 45, 58, 66 and 83-93 kDa. Results showing four positive bands, or five equivocal (borderline) bands, report as negative and are completely disregarded. Bands 31 kDa and 34 kDa—both of which are significant antigens that appear later in the immune response and are highly Lyme specific—so specific, in fact, that these bands represent the antigens used in developing the Lyme vaccine—are also excluded. How ironic that these antigens were relevant enough for developing the Lyme disease vaccine, but not relevant enough to be included in the laboratory reporting for Lyme. (By the way, the Lyme vaccine is no longer available due to numerous lawsuits by people who believed that the vaccine made them sick and actually infected them with Lyme disease; the manufacturer cites "low sales" as the reason for the withdrawal in 2002).

To demonstrate this, one study showed that although 89% of patients with EM rash developed IgG antibodies as detected by Western Blot some time during their disease, only 22% were positive by the standards of the CDC.[5]

Another limitation to the Western Blot is the CDC's belief that an IgM Western Blot should only be used within the first month of infection, even though other studies have shown that the IgM Western Blot can be positive even in recurrent or persistent disease. Some patients who have been ill for many years will still show a positive IgM Western Blot and a negative IgG Western Blot. Other patients with culture-positive Lyme disease will remain seronegative on any kind of Western Blot testing (approximately 20-30% in fact). Such is the challenge of Lyme disease testing.

Although the most clinically useful of all indirect tests, a positive Western Blot still only suggests exposure to Lyme disease, it does not diagnose Lyme disease. Diagnosis is still done based on the clinical picture—a person's history and exposure coupled with their current symptoms.

Testing for Co-Infections

Along with testing for Borrelia, it is imperative to test for co-infections. Information gained from co-infection testing can make a significant difference to the treatment path chosen. Different microbes require different medications and different herbs to counter them. Probably the best example of this is Babesia. Babesia is a parasite, while Borrelia is a bacterium. The medications that work well for Borrelia will not work well for Babesia. The consensus among hundreds of Lyme-treating doctors is that undetected and untreated co-infections are one of the key reasons for treatment failure in Lyme disease.

There are a few different ways to test for co-infections. The main types are antibody tests, FISH tests and PCR tests.

Antibody Tests

The co-infections that IGeneX offers antibody testing for are:

- Babesia duncani
- Babesia microti
- Bartonella species
- Ehrlichia chafeensis (HME)
- Anaplasma phagocytophila (HGA)
- Rickettsia rickettsii/ typhi

Antibody testing, similar to what we discussed in the indirect tests for Borrelia, measures the immune system's reaction to these various microbes. The tests done are IgG and IgM. Remember, IgM is a marker of either a new infection or current/ active infection. IgG indicates either prior exposure or a more chronic/ longer-term infection.

In interpreting these tests, I regard an elevation in either antibody clinically significant when combined with a symptomatic patient. IGeneX criteria for all the co-infections listed above are the following:

IgM	<20	negative
IgM	20-160	may or may not indicate active infection
IgM	>160	indicates an active infection
IgG	<40	negative
IgG	40-160	may or may not indicate active infection
IgG	>160	indicates an active infection

As an example, if a patient has an IgM level of 20 for a particular infection, I would consider treating that co-infection, *especially if the symptom picture matches that of the co-infection*. Remember, for co-infections as well as Borrelia, the diagnosis is based primarily on clinical presentation.

FISH Tests

The Fluorescent In-Situ Hybridization (FISH) test is a direct test—it does not rely on immune response and is a way to visualize the microbes directly—that uses a sample examined as a thin smear in order to identify and mark the ribosomal RNA. Under a microscope, the bugs, whose presence indicates an active, current infection, literally glow in the dark.

The Babesia FISH test detects both Babesia duncani and Babesia microti. It is performed on whole blood, since the parasites exist within the red blood cells themselves.

The Bartonella FISH test detects B. vinsonii, B. berkhoffii, B. henselae and B. quintana, so it can detect several different strains. The FISH test actually shows the microbes fluorescing under a microscope. Bartonella, rod-shaped bacteria, have been stained with a substance specific to mark them so a positive result will reflect the sighting of characteristic bacteria of this shape.

FISH tests have a high level of specificity so there are very few false positives. Remember though, a negative FISH does not necessarily mean that the infection is not present. It simply means that it was not detected in that particular sample.

PCR Tests

Like the FISH, PCR tests for co-infections are direct tests. DNA, or parts of the DNA of the bacteria, are evaluated in the blood sample. In my experience, FISH tests are more sensitive than PCR tests for co-infections and are more frequently utilized.

■ ■ ■ ■

By now you may be asking why we test at all, if the tests are not 100% reliable and if Lyme disease is a clinical diagnosis anyway. The answer is that the more information we can gather, the better. Testing can give confirmation on a suspected illness, shed light on which co-infections are present and help in assessing the severity of an infection. For example, if a patient tests indeterminate on the Lyme Western Blot but has a positive FISH test for Babesia and Babesia duncani antibodies at 80 or 160, then they may have a dominant Babesia infection, and treatment should start there.

Similarly, if a patient shows a positive PCR for Borrelia, a positive IgM Western Blot, and all negative co-infection testing, and unless they have symptoms that are pathognomonic of a specific co-infection, their initial treatment should be tailored around the Borrelia. However, another person can have positive antibodies to Borrelia, Babesia, Bartonella and Rickettsia, and in that case, we know we have a complex situation that is going to require several different medications to address them all.

Lab tests are very useful and should be regarded as important pieces of the puzzle. Alone, they do not rule in or out infection, but when combined with history, symptoms, tick exposures and so on can give very useful information to help shape the big picture.

■ ■ ■ ■

Other Tests That Might Be Useful

Not only are there tests for the infections themselves, but there are a couple of other markers and tests that can help assess an individual's health. This is not a complete list of tests as there are literally dozens of tests that may be useful in various scenarios.

CD-57

The CD-57 is not so much a test to detect Lyme disease as it is an immune marker that tends to be low in the presence of Lyme disease. CD, or cluster designation markers, are identifying markers on certain immune cells called T cells and NK cells. They give cells their variance in appearance and function. So far, there are approximately 200 known CD's, numbered according to their order of discovery. Any T cell or NK cell will carry many different CD markers.

If a cell expresses a certain marker, it is designated with the number of that marker and a "+" sign. So if an immune cell expresses the CD-57 marker, it is written as CD-57+. Through laboratory testing, we can measure the number of cells that carry a certain designation, either on the T cell or NK cell.

Clinically, measuring certain CD markers can help evaluate certain illnesses. Lyme disease has been associated with a low CD-57 count—specifically Borrelia infection (as opposed to co-infections). The sicker the patient, the lower the CD-57 count appears to be.

Measuring the CD-57 count can be helpful for a number of reasons. First, other illnesses such as chronic fatigue syndrome, rheumatoid arthritis or multiple sclerosis might mimic Lyme, but those illnesses will not cause a drop in the CD-57, so this marker can help in determining Lyme disease as distinct from other chronic illnesses with similar symptom pictures. Also, the CD-57 can be used to track treatment progress, as it should return towards normal levels as the infection improves. It also can give clues into co-infections. CD-57 levels are impacted by Borrelia but not significantly by co-infections, so if a patient is still symptomatic despite Lyme treatment and has a rising CD-57 count, it can be a clue that co-infections, not the Borrelia itself, are driving the remaining symptoms.

Of course, nothing is as straightforward as it seems, especially in Lyme disease. Many chronically ill Lyme patients present with a low CD-57 count, and despite long-term treatment and a resolving symptom picture, their counts stay frustratingly low. There are sometimes discrepancies between one lab and another, and numbers can fluctuate up and down between readings in ways that do not seem to correlate with the degree of illness or recovery.

It is important to remember that the lab is running the CD-57 on the NK cells, not the T cells. T cells will express CD-57 markers, but they are not clinically relevant to Lyme in the same way that the CD-57+ NK cells are. Running the CD-57 test on the T cells may be one reason for apparent discrepancies in results.

The CD-57 test is a worthwhile test to run as a gauge of immune response to Borrelia. While it sometimes shows inconsistencies, it may provide another piece of the puzzle and more information to shed light on that person's case. In the United States, the CD-57+ NK test is available through Labcorp as well as IGeneX.

Fry Labs Advanced Stain for Biofilm

We have already seen that the production of biofilm by colonies of bacteria can create bacterial defenses that are difficult to overcome. The bacterial colonies produce biofilm then hide in it, evading antibiotic and immune attack. The colonies become quite sophisticated—they attach to other structures that allow the flow of nutrients in and toxins out of their milieu, making them very resilient.

Fry Labs (Arizona, U.S.) initially began smear testing to provide assessment of Bartonella and other protozoans in the blood of chronically ill patients. As their work progressed, they saw colonies with biofilm in many of the blood samples. They have further developed their stain techniques and can provide insight into the degree of biofilm involvement, literally giving a visual picture of it. In patients who are being treated with antibiotic therapy and making slow or minimal progress, assessing biofilm may be of great value.

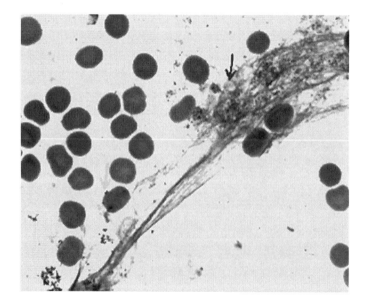

Demonstration of biofilm development on a smear test through Fry Laboratories[6]

Elispot-LTT (Lymphocyte Transformation Test)

Run by Infectolab in Augsburg, Germany, the Elispot-LTT test uses a different part of the immune system to the antibody testing. Antibodies are part of the humoral immune response; we also have a cellular immune response that involves T cells and NK cells (the CD-57 cell marker described above is part of the cellular immune system).

A Borrelia infection will activate T cells as well as antibodies. Activation of T cells occurs immediately after infection, and stops approximately six to eight weeks after completion of effective therapy or when the infection is resolved. Therefore, measuring T cell reactivity to Borrelia might be another useful diagnostic tool, as it is not as subject to the variability of antibody responses in different patients and at different times of infection.

According to Infectolab, the Elispot-LTT will detect even a single reactive T cell, is accurate in both acute and chronic infection, and is a helpful indicator of whether infection is truly resolved at the end of therapy. The Elispot-LTT test is available for a range of infectious agents including Borrelia, Chlamydia pneumonia, Chlamydia trachomatis, Ehrlichia, Anaplasma, Yersinia and the Epstein-Barr virus.

Infectolab
49-821-4550-740 (ph)
49-821-4550-741 (fax)
service@infectolab.de (email)
www.infectolab.de (website)

Inherent Challenges in Lyme Disease Testing

As you can see, there are several challenges to getting accurate and reliable testing for Lyme disease.

The first is that the ELISA test is the first test administered if Lyme is suspected. We have already seen that the ELISA test is not a sufficiently sensitive test to be clinically useful. Unfortunately, many doctors run the ELISA test, and if the results are negative, make a definitive statement that the person does not have Lyme disease. Any discussion of Lyme disease after that meets with cold response or total dismissal.

In those very few cases where the ELISA test comes back positive, a follow up confirmation test would be the Western Blot. If run through larger commercial labs, the Western Blot test is not going to recognize some of the bands that are necessary to give the complete picture, such as the 31 and 34 kDa bands.

Often, if an ELISA is negative, doctors will not run Western Blots at all. They have been taught about the two-tier testing—ELISA first, then Western Blot only if ELISA is positive. That two-tiered system was designed for research and epidemiological purposes; it was never meant to be used for clinical diagnostic purposes and is simply not appropriate or adequate in the clinical setting.

Any of the indirect tests have the inherent challenge that they measure immune response. We know that Lyme can dampen immune response, so the very markers needed to diagnose infection are dampened by the infection itself, leading to a lower chance of diagnosis. It is ironic that the more profound and chronic the infection in the body, the lesser the response may be on indirect testing.

Adequate testing for co-infections is often not performed. This leads to an incomplete picture of a person's chronic infections and may lead to inadequacies in treatment protocols.

Getting the Most Out of Laboratory Testing for Lyme Disease

There are ways to get more reliable and comprehensive testing done. Here are some ways to maximize laboratory information:

- Make sure testing is done through a lab that has expertise in Lyme and co-infection testing, and is not restricted to CDC criteria. IGeneX Laboratory in Palo Alto, California is a specialist Lyme lab that offers the most reliable and comprehensive testing at this time. It is possible to send blood samples from most countries to IGeneX via Fedex or other international courier.
- To run IGeneX testing, contact the lab directly and request a blood kit. A doctor's signature is required on the requisition form to authorize the testing.

IGeneX Laboratory

1-650-424-1191 (ph)

1-650-424-1196 (fax)

customerservice@igenex.com (email)

www.igenex.com (website)

- Run as many different types of tests as possible, both direct and indirect. This means doing IFA, PCR and Western Blots for Borrelia. IGeneX testing (PCR and Western Blot) also covers a variety of strains of Borrelia, including the B. afzilii, B. garinii, and B. andersonii, meaning it is relevant for strains found in other countries as well as North American strains.
- Based on the data that IGeneX has collected to date, a comprehensive Lyme panel will detect about 80% of all Lyme patients (this represents the sensitivity of the test). The overall specificity of this panel is greater than 95% with all three types of tests run (IFA, Western Blot and PCR).
- Always do co-infection testing in conjunction with Lyme testing. Co-infections often go undiagnosed, and that can contribute significantly to treatment failures. The IGeneX panels cover Babesia, Bartonella, Ehrlichia, Anaplasma and Rickettsia. Ideally, antibody and FISH tests (available for Babesia and Bartonella only) would be run. PCR testing is also available for co-infections.
- If there is poor response to antimicrobial therapy or if improvement is slow, consider that biofilm might be an issue. We will discuss ways to deal with biofilm in the treatment section, however one option for evaluation is through the Advanced Stain by Fry Laboratories.

Fry Laboratories

1-480-292-8560 (ph)

1-480-656-4932 (fax)

info@frylabs.com (email)

www.frylabs.com (website)

- To get as complete a picture as possible, run additional immune markers such as the CD-57 NK cell count. Make sure the lab uses the NK cells, not the T cells, in their testing methodology. C4a and C3a complement are two other markers that may indicate inflammation and neurotoxicity in the system. These are also immune markers that can be run through local, commercial labs.

- Determine whether antimicrobial therapy is indicated prior to testing. There are mixed views as to whether testing should be "provoked", that is, an antimicrobial given for a few weeks before the blood is collected with the aim of killing off some microbes and stirring up the immune system to produce a louder "noise" for the test to measure. Certainly, many patients are too ill to be able to tolerate such an approach, as the Herxheimer reaction may be too great (more on Herxheimer reactions in the following section). Many patients require a gentler introduction to antimicrobial therapy, whereas a provocation can require higher doses right off the bat. Also, many patients would have a difficult time convincing their local doctor to give them such doses of antibiotics without an official diagnosis to base it on.

Having said that, there are some cases where I have used antibiotics and/ or antimicrobial herbs to try to generate a greater immune response. And there are some cases where a negative IgM Western Blot has turned into a positive Western Blot after a few weeks of antimicrobial therapy. In general, I do not use provocation for the majority of my patients prior to testing.

The most important thing to stress is that Lyme disease is still a clinical diagnosis. We use lab testing to support that diagnosis, to give information on co-infections, and to give quantitative information that we can use over the course of treatment to track progress. The best way to get accurate and reliable information is to do testing through a specialty Lyme lab such as IGeneX and to run a variety of test types (both direct and indirect) to increase the likelihood of revealing evidence of the infection. Co-infection testing is imperative to round out the picture.

REFERENCES

1. Bakken LL, Callister SM, Wand PJ, Schell RF. Interlaboratory comparison of test results for detection of Lyme disease by 516 participants in the Wisconsin State laboratory of hygiene/College of American Pathologists proficiency testing program. J Clin Microbiol. 1997 Mar;35(3):537-43.

2. Engstrom SM, Shoop E, Johnson RC. Immunoblot interpretation criteria for serodiagnosis of early Lyme disease. J Clin Microbiol. 1995 Feb;33(2):419-27.

3. Aguero-Rosenfeld ME, Nowakowski J, McKenna DF, Carbonaro CA, Wormser GP. Serodiagnosis in early Lyme disease. J Clin Microbiol. 1993 Dec;31(12):3090-3095.

4. Aguero-Rosenfeld ME, Nowakowski J, McKenna DF, Carbonaro CA, Wormser GP. Evolution of the serologic response to Borrelia burgdorferi in treated patients with culture-confirmed erythema migrans. J Clin Microbiol. 1996 Jan;34(1):l-9.

5. Aguero-Rosenfeld ME, Nowakowski J, McKenna DF, Carbonaro CA, Wormser GP. Evolution of the serologic response to Borrelia burgdorferi in treated patients with culture-confirmed erythema migrans. J Clin Microbiol. 1996 Jan;34(1):l-9.

6. Patient sample, reproduced with permission.

SECTION THREE

TREATMENT GUIDELINES FOR LYME DISEASE

Lyme disease is a multi-factorial and multi-system illness. It affects many different body systems, from immune function to hormones, and it creates a wide range of different symptoms. Any treatments undertaken, whether pharmaceutical or naturopathic, must address these multiple facets.

Chronic Lyme disease is not an easy illness to treat. There are several major considerations when creating treatment protocols for Lyme disease.

Please note: The treatment guidelines contained in this book are for informational purposes only; they are not intended to be prescriptions for treatment for any individual or individuals. Consult a licensed, qualified physician before attempting to use any Lyme disease treatment. Use of the treatment guidelines in this book while not under the care of a licensed physician may result in injury or death. Your own licensed physician should be the one to make final decisions about your medical care and which treatments you use.

11. TREATMENT CONSIDERATIONS

Treatment consideration #1:

Lyme disease may require hefty doses of antibiotics for a long time

The first point to know is that the bacteria and parasites in Lyme disease often require higher than typical doses of certain antibiotic and antiparasitic medications. A good example is doxycycline. Doxycycline is often dosed at 100mg twice daily but in Lyme disease, research has shown that dose to be bacteriostatic—that is, it will halt the progression of the bacteria but not fully kill it off. To be bacteriocidal, or able to fully kill the bacteria, Borrelia requires doses of 400mg per day. This is alarming to some doctors who have not prescribed doses that high in the past, and some patients have been denied treatment for this reason.

Yes, Lyme disease requires multiple antibiotics at high doses. It is part of what makes it a challenging illness to treat. I will discuss how to prevent side effects and protect the body during these long courses of antibiotics in the section on naturopathic treatments.

The duration of treatment is also a contentious one, due to the IDSA guidelines, which list 28 days as the longest duration of treatment, even in severe neurological Lyme. In reality, chronic Lyme disease requires far longer treatment times than that. The average treatment time for most patients is from 12-24 months. I rarely see a patient who can resolve their symptoms in less than 12 months. Some require 2-3 years of treatment; and yet others fare best when they continue with some kind of antibiotic protocol indefinitely.

A rule of thumb that is followed by many Lyme-literate medical doctors operating under ILADS protocols is to treat for two months beyond resolution of a person's symptoms. That means that a person must feel like they have been back to their old self (if they can remember what that is!) for a couple of months before discontinuing antibiotics. Even then, it is sensible to continue with herbal antimicrobials for a few months beyond ceasing antibiotics, to further address any remaining infection and to prevent relapse.

Treatment consideration #2:

Treatment must be a multi-tiered, multi-layered approach

We have already seen that chronic Lyme disease involves an infection with the Borrelia bacteria, and that Borrelia can exist in three different forms—as a spirochete, a cell-wall deficient form and a cyst form. The bacteria can morph back and forth between forms to evade attack by the immune system and antimicrobial therapy.

Each form of Borrelia is susceptible to different antibiotics. *Therefore each of the three forms must be addressed for recovery to be possible.* If only one form of Borrelia is treated, it can simply morph into other forms and long-term improvement will be elusive.

Even for Borrelia in the absence of co-infections, three medications must be layered into the treatment protocol—one for spirochetes, one for cell-wall deficient forms, and one for cyst forms. In some cases, natural treatments can be substituted for medications, but by and large, three antibiotics are required.

Typically, the medications are commenced one at a time, spaced out by 2-4 weeks to allow the body time to adjust to one before adding another. This also allows time to gauge any allergic or other medication reactions without confusing which one is the culprit. Ultimately, the goal is to have coverage of the three different forms.

We have also seen that Lyme disease often involves different microbes known as co-infections, including Bartonella, Babesia, Ehrlichia and

Rickettsia. Mycoplasma is another common microbe in Lyme patients. These co-infections must also be addressed in addition to the Borrelia. When the co-infections are bacterial in nature, it is easier to do this, as there may be crossover benefit between Lyme medications and medications that will be effective for the co-infection. Examples are doxycycline and minocycline, both of which are used for Borrelia, Mycoplasma and Ehrlichia. Babesia, on the other hand, is a tougher case because it is an intra-cellular parasite. The medications that are effective for Borrelia will not be effective for Babesia since one is a bacteria and the other is a parasite. Babesia will require its own medication protocol.

Part of the challenge is deciphering where to start. This is where lab work can come in very handy. If a particular infection is registering very high antibodies, then likely it is a potent infection that requires prioritizing. If a patient has a strongly positive Western Blot that shows activity in several different bands and a mild elevation of Bartonella antibodies, the Borrelia appears dominant, and I would consider starting there. Treating Lyme disease can be compared to peeling layers off an onion, and it must be determined which layer of the onion is currently the top layer, and should be dealt with first.

If Babesia is present, it moves up the priority list to number one, especially when the patient's symptoms reflect a Babesia infection because Babesia is a very disruptive infection, and progress against the other infections will most likely be out of reach until it is addressed. The symptoms I look for in Babesia include night sweats, low-grade fevers, temperature regulation problems, neck pain, head and neck symptoms such as ringing in the ears and blurry vision, spaciness and feeling "detached," and complete hormonal mayhem. Flushing in the face, mottling of the skin anywhere on the body, and tiny red dots on the skin called capillary angiomas are also clues.

A person presenting with more neurological issues such as cognitive deficits, numbness and tingling in any part of the body, Bell's palsy, along with joint and muscle pain that migrates, suggests a dominant Borrelia infection. A patient with agonizing pain in the soles of their feet, where it feels like walking on glass in the morning, rib pain, severe anxiety and weird looking scratches or stretch marks on their skin may have Bartonella.

Typically we start with what seems to be the dominant infection. Babesia, if suspected, is given high priority in treatment as an ongoing Babesia infection can hinder progress of Lyme treatment. We also adjust treatment protocols based on the patient's response. If a patient is getting treated primarily for one infection with limited benefit, it may be that a co-infection is present and creating most of that person's symptoms. In general, co-infections hinder progress against Borrelia.

Treatment consideration #3:

There might be Herxheimer reactions

The third factor to consider when shaping Lyme treatment is the possibility of Herxheimer reactions (or Jarisch-Herxheimer reaction), aka "Herxes." Adolf Jarisch, an Austrian dermatologist, and Karl Herxheimer, a German dermatologist, put their names to these reactions when they discovered the phenomena while treating syphilis with mercury back in the late 1800s and early 1900s. Today, "Herxing" has become just as valid a verb as "googling," especially in the Lyme community.

Herxing refers to a temporary worsening of symptoms, caused by the release of neurotoxins as pathogens are killed. It is the pathogens themselves that release the neurotoxins, but it becomes the task of the body to detoxify and excrete them. Herxing typically reflects a transient worsening of a person's existing symptoms, or even the onset of new symptoms.

While spirochetes are renowned for their ability to trigger Herxes, other bacteria such as Bartonella can, too. I have also observed significant Herx reactions in patients with Candida (yeast) overgrowth when it is treated, and also in the parasitic illness Babesia.

Inherent in these die-off reactions is an elevation in cytokines, which are chemical mediators of the immune system. Some cytokines will lessen symptoms and moderate inflammation, while some will kick it up. The cytokines involved in Herxes are more inflammatory, and therefore will give the patient the experience of a worsening of symptoms, and possibly even the introduction of new symptoms.

The body works hard to clear the endotoxins that have been released, through its natural detoxification mechanisms. Variations in a patient's experience of Herxing depend greatly on their detoxification mechanisms. Many people with chronic Lyme disease have compromised detoxification systems, which makes the Herxheimer reactions more profound. Primary detoxification mechanisms include the liver, kidneys, and skin.

There are ways to assist the body in detoxifying the toxins that arise in a Herx reaction, and those will be discussed under naturopathic therapies. For now, suffice it to say that treating Lyme disease may well lead to Herxheimer reactions, and it is important to be aware of them. Different people will have different levels of sensitivity to the endotoxins released by dying organisms. For some, it is possible to push through Herxes and continue treatment. For others, the pace of treatment may be dictated by the severity of the Herxes. If Herxes get too severe, treatment will need to be slowed or even stopped for a period of time for the patient to stabilize. Herxing is not a "badge of honor" where how much they can endure proves how tough they are. There are some times where Herxing can in fact be dangerous for the individual.

Herxing is also not required for the treatment to work. Some people do not Herx significantly at all when starting treatment and still benefit from the treatment, usually those who are genetically good detoxifiers, pay attention to their nutrition, and supplement with supportive nutrients and herbs for detoxification. This may also be the case during treatment of early or uncomplicated infection.

Herxing is not limited to pharmaceutical protocols. Antibiotics and natural treatment modalities can both cause Herxes. Additionally, Rifing —a frequency-based therapy, Hyperbaric Oxygen Therapy (HBOT), and other antibacterial treatments can all trigger the Herxheimer reaction. Effectively, anything that kills off these bugs can trigger Herxes.

It can be tricky to determine whether a patient is having a Herx reaction or an adverse reaction to a particular antibiotic, but I have two guidelines for this:

1. A medication reaction is usually quite immediate—within minutes to hours of taking the drug. A Herxheimer reaction often takes several days to appear (as the endotoxins build up gradually and reach a tipping point at which stage they make the person feel worse).

2. A medication reaction often produces new symptoms, and/or shows up as allergy-type symptoms such as nausea, headaches and rashes. A Herxheimer reaction is typically representative of the symptoms the person usually experiences, just in a more severe way, so there may be more joint pain, more cognitive deficits, more night sweats—whatever the person's usual symptoms are, but flared. Often people have an intuitive sense of whether a worsening of symptoms is a medication reaction or a Herx reaction.

It can also be tricky deciding whether to push through a Herx or slow down treatment to let the body recover and catch up. Some guidelines for this include:

1. The person's lifestyle—Do they have to work to support themselves? Do they have someone to care for them at home? How functional do they need to be in their daily lives? An example might be a college-age person who has the summer off and wants to use that time to treat aggressively. They may be willing to go through more severe Herxing to get through it within a set time frame. A single Mom who has to work to support her family is more likely to need a slow and steady approach.

2. Any life-threatening aspects to the Herxes—Some patients with motor neuron disease may have breathing or swallowing difficulties so a Herx reaction could be life threatening. Severe cardiac involvement is another questionable symptom. If a patient has major tachycardia or arrhythmia, pushing too much can be dangerous.

Herxing can be a significant phenomenon and can greatly impact the pace at which treatment progresses. Often, awareness of what Herxing is and what can be expected goes a long way towards alleviating the anxiety that may be caused by symptoms seemingly getting worse at the start of treatment. I always assure my patients that some Herx reaction is to be expected, that the "worse before better" is typical, and may even be a good sign that the treatment is working well. But I also monitor them closely and will advise people to back off or slow down a particular medication or therapy if I feel that their body is not keeping up with the die-off reactions produced. The patient's safety must always come first; then their need to be functional in their daily lives and their psycho-emotional capacity to withstand Herxing should be closely considered.

Treatment consideration #4:

What works for one might not work for another

There is a great individualization of treatment that must take place in addressing Lyme disease. An obvious factor in this is medication allergies. A person with a penicillin allergy is not going to be able to take a medication that a non-allergic person can take, and alternative medications will need to be chosen.

Medication side effects can drive treatment decisions. One of the side effects of doxycycline is sun sensitivity. Some people may experience that side effect so severely that they just cannot take doxycycline. Nausea, vomiting, headaches, tinnitus, and many other side effects may present themselves. Even within medication classes, two very slightly different drugs may give totally different side effects, for example, azithromycin and clarithromycin, both in the macrolide family. One person might tolerate one well, and the other not at all. Another patient might be the exact opposite.

Remember, medication allergies and side effects are different from Herxheimer reactions, which we often discern as a worsening of the person's usual symptoms.

In some cases, different people simply benefit more from one medication choice or combination than another. To some extent this can be predicted (especially by co-infection picture), but sometimes it appears to have no rhyme or reason. The reality is medication protocols can at times seem like trial and error. There is no guarantee that what works for one person will work equally well for another. Often, treatment decisions have to be made one at a time, step-by-step, depending on the reaction to the last step, and adjusted along the way wherever necessary. Awareness and understanding of this can make the treatment journey much less frustrating.

Treatment consideration #5:

Plateaus may occur with long-term antibiotic use

If a medication is continued for a long duration, the pathogens may become resistant to it, and the medication will lose its desired effect. To overcome this, medications should be rotated periodically. The time frame may vary—Dr. Joseph Burrascano suggests every six weeks. My rule of thumb in clinical practice is to continue medication regardless of duration of treatment as long as the patient is improving. If the patient has hit a plateau and is clearly not improving on that regimen, I will change the protocol. Typically one medication will be changed at a time so as not to overwhelm the patient's system or trigger another major Herx from too many new medications. Also, the choice of which new drugs to add into the mix should take into account which infections are currently dominant, or on the "top" layer of the onion that we are trying to "peel."

12. SUGGESTED MEDICATION PROTOCOLS

THERE IS NO COOKIE-CUTTER, ONE-SIZE-FITS-ALL PROTOCOL FOR Lyme disease treatment, but there are certain guidelines and plans that make sense. Let us now turn to the various medications that can be used to address these different infections. Please note that the following treatment protocols have been drawn from the ILADS treatment guidelines, Dr. Joseph Burrascano's Treatment Guidelines, information presented by other Lyme-literate medical doctors and experts in the field at ILADS conferences, and my own clinical experience. This information does not represent the position of the IDSA, which believes only in 14-28 days of antibiotic therapy. I believe their position is flawed and not valid in the real world of Lyme disease.

Acute, or Early Stage, Lyme Disease

Before we go through all the various medications used in chronic Lyme treatment, let us look at possible medication protocols for acute Lyme. Acute Lyme here refers to the first few weeks of infection. As we have learned, lab testing may not be reliable at that early stage as the immune system may not yet have mounted a response, so diagnosis is made based on history of tick bite, EM rash and/ or flu-like illness following a tick exposure.

If a person has had a known tick bite, it may be indicated to do prophylactic treatment even in the absence of the EM rash or symptoms. It is critical to begin treatment as quickly as possible in early Lyme disease, as early, aggressive treatment may prevent the development of chronic Lyme disease and may literally save the patients' quality of life for years to come.

A prophylactic protocol could involve four weeks of the following combination of antibiotics:

> Doxycycline 200mg—twice daily
> Tinidazole 500mg—twice daily

Western Blot testing would be done 6-8 weeks after the bite.

For a known acute Lyme illness, 6-8 weeks of treatment is required, but if treated early enough and aggressively enough, Lyme may be eradicated completely. Doxycycline is typically the medication of choice in early Lyme, not only because of its activity against Borrelia but also for its ability to eliminate Ehrlichia and some of the other co-infections.

The following is Dr. Richard Horowitz's acute Lyme protocol (presented at ILADS Conference, Toronto, 2011)[1]:

First month:
> Doxycycline 200mg—twice daily
> Hydroxychloroquine (Plaquenil)—200mg twice daily; *or*
> Tinidazole 500mg—twice daily

Second month:
> Cefuroxime 500mg—twice daily
> Azithromycin 500mg—once daily; or clarithromycin 500mg –twice daily
> Hydroxychloroquine (Plaquenil) - 200mg twice daily; *or*
> Tinidazole - 500mg twice daily

I have also combined the following and prescribed a two-month protocol of:
> Doxycycline 200mg—twice daily
> Azithromycin 500mg—once daily
> Cefuroxime 500mg—three times daily
> Tinidazole 500mg—twice daily

If the person is not symptomatic at the end of the two-month protocol, it is still advised to follow with antimicrobial herbs for two more months. If no symptoms remain beyond that, Lyme disease has probably been eradicated. If symptoms persist, however, treatment would be continued per the regimens for chronic Lyme disease.

Chronic Lyme Treatment

For simplicity and organization of information, the medication protocols suggested are listed according to which phase of the Borrelia life cycle they address, or for the intended co-infection.

BORRELIA

Spirochete forms of Borrelia

The medications used for these forms act by damaging the spirochete's cell wall. The two main classes of medications are penicillins and cephalosporins, although work by Eva Sapi of University of New Haven indicates that tinidazole (listed here under cyst-form medications below) may be an effective medication for all forms of Lyme disease including spirochete forms.[2]

Penicillins

Amoxicillin:

Amoxicillin is an oral form of penicillin. It is not considered the most effective antibiotic for Borrelia, but amoxicillin is still more effective than penicillin V. High doses ranging from 3-6 grams per day must be taken to achieve benefit.

To boost the effectiveness of amoxicillin, probenecid can be given simultaneously, at a dose of 500mg every 8 hours. Another alternative is Augmentin XR, which is amoxicillin and clavulanate. 1000mg can be given every 8 hours, up to 2000mg every 12 hours. Additional amoxicillin may still have to be given separately for full benefit.

Amoxicillin is contraindicated in anyone with a penicillin allergy. It can be safely used in pregnancy and breastfeeding, and is often given to children.

Bicillin LA:

Bicillin LA is given as an injection into the muscle, administered 2-3 times per week. It is a long-acting penicillin so it is easier to get sustained levels of this antibiotic, which gives greater benefit. Bicillin LA is significantly more effective than oral amoxicillin due to its good central nervous system penetration, which helps neurological symptoms. In particular, I find Bicillin LA to be very helpful in addressing the cognitive deficits that are so typical in Lyme disease, such as brain fog and memory loss. As an injectable, it bypasses the gastrointestinal tract so it does not contribute to gut issues to the same extent that oral antibiotics might.

As with oral amoxicillin, it should not be used in anyone with a penicillin allergy. Some patients find the injections themselves to be quite uncomfortable, and this can be partially offset by making sure the liquid is at room temperature before injecting (not straight out of the fridge) and by injecting it slowly, over a period of a few minutes. Heating pads afterwards can help disperse the medication through the muscle tissue, minimizing aching in the area.

I consider Bicillin LA to be a good compromise between oral and IV antibiotics. It comes in vials containing 1.2 million units. Most start with 1 vial injected in the gluteus muscle weekly, building up to three times weekly.

Bicillin injections can produce significant and prolonged Herxes. Some patients will notice a Herx reaction in the first few days while others experience it around day 25-30 of their Bicillin regimen. Bicillin LA is one of my favorite medications in the treatment of chronic Lyme disease.

Cephalosporins
Ceftriaxone:

Ceftriaxone is a 3rd generation cephalosporin that is given intravenously for the treatment of Lyme disease. Theoretically it can also be given intramuscularly, however that is not a practical long-term dosing method and is not widely used.

IV ceftriaxone has historically been given in doses of two grams every day. More recently, better results have been seen with pulsed dosing of two grams twice daily, four days on with three days off each week.

(See below for more information on the merits of IV versus oral antibiotics).

Cefuroxime axetil:

Cefuroxime axetil is a 2nd generation oral cephalosporin, and it is widely available. The recommended dose is 1 gram twice daily. Cefuroxime can be used during pregnancy and breastfeeding, and can be given to children.

In general, while 3rd generation cephalosporins are considered more effective than 1st and 2nd, cefuroxime has great benefit as it also has activity against Staph, so it is good for treating atypical EM rashes that may contain bacteria other than Borrelia.

Cell-wall deficient forms of Borrelia

Macrolides
Erythromycin:

This is not an effective medication for Borrelia and is not recommended.

Azithromycin:

Azithromycin is a gentle medication that is typically well tolerated. While it is not among the most effective for Borrelia itself nor used as a first-line therapy, it has its place in Lyme treatment protocols. I choose it as a starting medication in patients who have high sensitivity levels to pre-scription medications, sometimes dosing it just three days per week. It is more effective for musculoskeletal symptoms such as joint and muscle pain than neurological symptoms. Some individuals who would not be able to tolerate doxycycline can handle azithromycin. Typical doses are

500-600mg daily given in a single dose. Azithromycin has a very long half-life so once daily dosing is possible.

Clarithromycin:

Somewhat more potent and more effective than azithromycin, clarithromycin also has greater tolerability issues. Many people experience some gastrointestinal side effects such as nausea, as well as a metallic taste in the mouth. Clarithromycin may cause more significant Candida overgrowth problems when compared with azithromycin, in part because it must be dosed more frequently due to its shorter half-life.

Azithromycin and clarithromycin are not considered first line drugs for Lyme due to their limited effectiveness. This may relate to the fluid pocket created around the Borrelia bacteria in the cell. The fluid is quite acidic, meaning it has a low pH, and that acidity may inactivate azithromycin and clarithromycin. A way to overcome this is to give hydroxychloroquine (Plaquenil) or amantadine, which can raise the pH of the fluid and allow the two medications to work better. (This does not apply to telithromycin, which is not affected by the pH levels).

In spite of their limitations, azithromycin and clarithromycin still have a significant place in Lyme disease therapy especially when combined with other antibiotics. They are just not stand-alone medications. Mepron, a medication for Babesia, requires either azithromycin or clarithromycin for it to work effectively, so sometimes that dictates the inclusion of such medications in an individual's protocol. Also, azithromycin and clarithromycin, having the same purpose as the tetracyclines such as doxycycline and minocycline (which is to target cell-wall deficient forms), tend to work well along with them. They act slightly differently as they work on slightly different ribosomes, but they fulfil the same goal and are often used concurrently for that reason.

Clindamycin:

Clindamycin is sometimes used for Borrelia and also Bartonella. It can be effective as it penetrates the central nervous system and gets deep into other tissues to address deep-seated infection in the body. The biggest caution with clindamycin is its propensity to cause pseudomembranous colitis, which will cause unrelenting diarrhea. Prevention is the key with high doses of mixed strain probiotics including Saccharomyces boulardii. The dose of clindamycin is 300mg two to three times daily.

Telithromycin:

Telithromycin, although not widely used, may be the most effective of the macrolide antibiotics. It has more serious side effects such as cardiac irregularities and liver enzyme elevation, so it requires close monitoring (EKG and liver enzymes every two weeks). It also has numerous interactions with other medications due to its effect on liver enzyme systems that regulate the metabolism of certain drugs. Telithromycin can provoke strong and prolonged Herxheimer reactions. It is dosed at 800mg once daily, and does not need amantadine or hydroxychloroquine to boost its efficacy. Given its toxicity and side effect profile, many Lyme-literate medical doctors in the United States will not prescribe telithromycin.

Tetracyclines

Doxycycline:

Doxycycline is perhaps the most widely used medication in Lyme disease treatment. It is used in acute Lyme but is equally effective in more chronic cases. Doxycycline has broad-spectrum activity against Borrelia along with co-infections such as Bartonella, Ehrlichia and Mycoplasma.

Doses of doxycycline are typically 200mg twice daily and as high as 600mg daily. 200mg twice daily has been shown to be more effective than 100mg four times daily. It should not to be used during pregnancy or breastfeeding, or in children younger than eight years of age (it can cause irreversible tooth staining in kids). Side effects of doxycycline include headaches, gastrointestinal disturbance and increased sun sensitivity. It is best taken two hours away from metronidazole and tinidazole due to its ability to bind with them and impede absorption, and also two hours away from dairy products and minerals such as calcium and magnesium.

It has a broader spectrum of activity than minocycline when addressing Lyme with co-infections.

<u>Minocycline:</u>

Minocycline is not used as widely as doxycycline in Lyme disease treatment. It is more lipid soluble than doxycycline so it may have greater benefit in neuroborreliosis, but for this same reason it tends to have more vestibular side effects such as headache and dizziness. The dosing of minocycline is 100mg three times daily. It creates slightly less sun sensitivity and GI side effects as compared with doxycycline, but despite this, doxycycline remains the preferred choice. Minocycline is sometimes used for its profound anti-inflammatory effects, which can be particularly helpful in reducing neurological symptoms.

<u>Tetracycline:</u>

Tetracycline dosed at 500mg three to four times daily may be used if well tolerated. It is not used as frequently as minocycline or doxycycline, perhaps due to its lower central nervous system penetration or tolerability issues.

Cyst forms of Borrelia

<u>Metronidazole (Flagyl):</u>

Metronidazole can be used for cyst forms of Borrelia but has gastrointestinal side effects and tolerability issues. For this reason it is not my first choice. It is dosed 500mg twice daily and can be pulsed 2 weeks on/ 2 weeks off. Optimally it is dosed separately from doxycycline or minocycline by two hours.

Metronidazole is not safe in pregnancy as it can cause birth defects, but it can be used in children. Metronidazole will heighten one's sensitivity to alcohol and cause severe reactions, so patients on metronidazole are warned to avoid all alcohol. Since herbal tinctures are often preserved with alcohol, more sensitive patients put their herbs in hot water to evaporate off the alcohol before drinking them. For most patients the amount of alcohol in drop doses of herbs will not be enough to cause them problems.

Tinidazole:

Tinidazole comes with many of the same cautions as metronidazole, as it is in the same family of drugs. It cannot be used in pregnancy and does not combine well with alcohol, yet tinidazole seems to be much better tolerated and causes less GI upset. The dosing schedule is the same—500mg twice daily, pulsed two weeks on/ two weeks off. Tinidazole is my first choice in cyst-form medications for Borrelia. As with metronidazole, it can provoke quite significant Herxes, however most notice that after the first two or three cycles, the Herx reaction is lessened. Professor Eva Sapi studied metronidazole and tinidazole and found that the latter was much more effective in destroying colonies of Borrelia.

Plaquenil:

Plaquenil is essentially an anti-malaria drug, although it has multiple uses in medicine. In Lyme treatment we primarily use it to address cyst forms of Borrelia.

Plaquenil is widely used by rheumatologists for Rheumatoid Arthritis. It has anti-inflammatory effects, and appears to have immune modulating effects. I have found that Plaquenil can lessen pain and inflammation in Lyme patients with severe musculoskeletal symptoms. Unlike prednisone, which is immune suppressive *(and should never be used in patients with Lyme),* Plaquenil is more immune modulating and balancing, thus reducing the autoimmune process without wiping out the beneficial and necessary parts of immune function.

Another benefit of Plaquenil as mentioned above is the way it can shift the pH of the cell to make azithromycin and clarithromycin work better.

One of the major cautions with Plaquenil is that long-term use can cause retinal artery problems. Patients are advised to get an eye exam before starting treatment and every three months thereafter.

Alinia:

Alinia has less of a track record in chronic Lyme disease treatment but in recent years has been used as a cyst-form medication. It may also be effective for Babesia, thus having double benefit. The dosage is 500mg twice daily. Alinia's on-label use is intestinal parasitic infections such as Giardia and Cryptosporidium, and some patients do find that they have some diarrhea when starting Alinia. It is unclear whether that is medication sensitivity or a response to the die-off of existing intestinal parasites, although new research indicates that Lyme disease may in fact involve various parasitic infestations of not just the intestinal tract, but also other areas throughout the body.

REFERENCES

1. Horowitz RI. Lyme Disease & Babesiosis: updates on diagnosis and treatment 2011 [Video]. ILADS, producers. Toronto (CA): ILADS Conference; 2011. 10:58 min., sound, color. Available from: http://www.ilads.org/media/videos/videos_horowitz.php.

2. Sapi E, Kaur N, Anyanwu S, et al. Evaluation of in-vitro antibiotic susceptibility of different morphological forms of Borrelia burgdorferi. Infection and Drug Resistance [Internet]. 2011 [cited 2012 May];4:97-113. Available from: http://www.dovepress.com/evaluation-of-in-vitro-antibiotic-susceptibility-of-different-morpholo-peer-reviewed-article-IDR-MVP DOI: http://dx.doi.org/10.2147/IDR.S19201

13. MEDICATION PROTOCOLS
FOR CO-INFECTIONS

Babesia

Of all the co-infections, Babesia has the most distinct regimen of medications because it is a protozoal parasitic infection, not a bacterial infection as are Borrelia, Bartonella and Ehrlichia. Until recent years, the usual treatment regimen was clindamycin plus quinine; however, this regimen has been abandoned due to the unacceptable incidence of severe side effects.

Mepron (Atovaquone):

One of the primary medications of choice for Babesia, atovaquone goes under the brand name of Mepron in the United States. Nicknamed "liquid gold", mostly because of its price, it has a good track record in Babesia treatment. Standard dosage is 750mg twice daily, which equates to 1 teaspoon twice daily, however some patients need higher doses, up to 2 teaspoons twice daily. Atovaquone can cause a mild yellowish discoloration of the vision and mild gastrointestinal side effects but is generally quite well tolerated.

An important point about atovaquone is that it must be taken with significant amounts of fatty food to facilitate its absorption. Research shows that 22 grams of fat is the ideal amount. There are healthy ways to get this amount of fat without justifying a large helping of fries or a burger. See Appendix B for a list of healthy fats and fatty foods.

Atovaquone in the form of Mepron must be combined with a macrolide such as azithromycin, clarithromycin or telithromycin, in the standard dosages listed previously. Patients on Mepron should not take supplements containing CoQ10 or milk thistle, as those two supplements can reduce the efficacy of the Mepron.

When Babesia is chronic, at least four to six months of treatment is required. Multiple medications are often needed, as it can be a difficult infection to eradicate. Babesia duncani may be more aggressive and treatment resistant than Babesia microti.

Malarone:

Malarone is a combination of atovaquone and proguanil. Although the standard dose of Malarone contains only 1000mg of actual atovaquone compared with 1500mg in 10 mL of Mepron, the proguanil helps to boost its effectiveness. Malarone is dosed at 2 tablets twice daily of the 250/100mg strength. It does not need a macrolide antibiotic along with it (azithromycin/ clarithromycin), so may be a better starting point in more sensitive patients. When cost is a major issue, Malarone is marginally less expensive than Mepron. Both need high amounts of fatty foods taken at the same time to help with absorption. Overall, I consider Mepron to be a more potent medication than Malarone; concurrent use of Bactrim DS or Septra may boost its efficacy. CoQ10 and milk thistle should also be avoided when taking Malarone.

Lariam (Mefloquine):

Mefloquine is another medication that is used in malaria treatment and prophylaxis. It is a tablet dosed at 250mg once every five to seven days. It can be taken along with atovaquone. I typically use atovaquone for six to eight weeks to reduce the overall parasitic load before introducing mefloquine, however I have seen mefloquine be very effective on the neurological aspects of Babesia such as anxiety and depression.

Mefloquine carries with it some possible neuropsychiatric side effects. On the milder end, vivid dreams or an exacerbation of depression or anxiety may occur; on the more serious end, hallucinations, suicidal ideation and even psychosis have been reported.

My experience with mefloquine in my patients is that it can definitely cause a temporary worsening of psycho-emotional symptoms; however I have observed that to be consistent with a Herxheimer-type pattern where a patient's existing symptoms flare up at the beginning of treatment. I have not seen any cases of the more severe psychiatric side effects. Individuals with a history of bipolar disorder, schizophrenia or other serious mental illness would be poor candidates for mefloquine, but I consider it a very effective medication in Babesia treatment, particularly where Babesia is affecting the brain and causing psycho-emotional symptoms.

Coartem/ Riamet:

Under brand names of either Coartem or Riamet, these medications are a combination of artemether and lumefantrine. Again, they are used in malaria treatment, as well as Babesiosis. The advantage of Coartem is that it is only dosed twice a day for three days each month. The down side is that other Babesia medications and macrolide or quinolone antibiotics must be stopped for those three days plus two to three days on each side, so that can create quite a disruption in the overall treatment protocol.

Alinia:

Alinia has already been discussed as a possible cyst-form medication for Borrelia, but it also used in the treatment of Babesia. Dosing is 500mg twice daily. Alinia does not have as much of an established track record for Babesia as atovaquone, however I often use it in combination therapy, when either atovaquone ceases to have beneficial effect or the cost becomes prohibitive.

Septra/ Bactrim:

These two medications are a combination of trimethoprim and sulfamethoxazole. They are referred to as sulfa drugs, so anyone with an allergy to sulfa drugs cannot take either of these two medications.

Septra and Bactrim are good choices in combination therapy where Borrelia and co-infections are present. Subsequently I will choose these especially for treatment protocols for Borrelia along with the co-infections of Babesia or Bartonella. Significant Herxheimer reactions can be expected, sometimes lasting several weeks.

Bartonella

Rifampin:

Rifampin is one of the primary medications used in the treatment of Bartonella. It is not particularly effective for Borrelia but is a good medication to be used in combination therapy.

Rifampin may cause a harmless orange discoloration of urine, and even sweat and tears. This is due to the inherent color of the medication and not liver problems, as some people assume. Having said that, rifampin can be liver toxic, so liver enzymes must be monitored regularly (at least monthly).

Rifampin combines well with doxycycline for Bartonella treatment. Azithromycin and clarithromycin may increase its action and are commonly used along with it. In some cases, through influence on liver enzyme systems, it can impact the rate of metabolism of other drugs, so interactions should be monitored closely. Theoretically rifampin can be given with Mepron or Malarone, but it may reduce their efficacy. Dosing is 300mg twice daily, but is often commenced at 150mg twice daily to monitor sensitivity and Herx reactions.

Rifampin can cause hormone dysregulation including an increase in Sex Hormone Binding Globulin (SHBG), so people with hormone irregularities should be monitored closely or should not use Rifampin.

Septra/ Bactrim:

As in Babesia treatment, Septra or Bactrim DS can add a powerful boost to co-infection treatment protocols and both have been used in the treatment of Bartonella. See the section above on Babesia treatment for more information about these drugs.

Levaquin:

Levaquin is in the quinolone category of antibiotics (the same family as Ciprofloxacin). Dosing of Levaquin is 500-750mg daily.

Levaquin can be effective for Bartonella, but it is not my first choice due to its significant potential side effect of causing tendonitis, and even tendon rupture. Tendons are the connective tissues that connect bones to muscles, and tendonitis is the inflammation of these structures. Pain and swelling at the site are the primary signs, although in some cases rupture has occurred spontaneously, requiring surgical repair. Typically the larger tendons are affected first, such as the Achilles tendon behind the ankle, and tendons in the elbows and knees. Levaquin must be stopped at the first sign of tendon pain, although the risk of inflammation and even rupture may continue for several weeks or months. Preloading with magnesium may prevent issues, and high dose magnesium and vitamin C may be used to relieve pain and inflammation should it occur.

Other medications in this family are gemifloxacin (Factive) and moxifloxacin (Avalox).

Because of the tendon issue, the preferred choice of medications for Bartonella is a combination of doxycycline, rifampin and azithromycin. Septra/ Bactrim DS may be added in patients who are not allergic to sulfa drugs.

Ehrlichia/ Anaplasma and Rickettsia

Doxycycline:

Given in similar doses to Borrelia, doxycycline is effective against both Ehrlichia and Anaplasma. Higher doses over several months are typically required for chronic cases—400-600mg per day.

Rifampin:

In treatment failures with doxycycline, or in combination therapy, rifampin is the next medication of choice. 300mg twice daily is the dose, similar to Bartonella.

Mycoplasma

The role of Mycoplasma in tick-borne illness is not fully understood, but many Lyme patients are also infected with Mycoplasma.

Treatment regimens for Mycoplasma involve combination therapy using doxycycline or minocycline, hydroxychloroquine, and azithromycin. Rifampin or Septra can also be helpful. In cases that do not respond to these medications, a quinolone such as Levaquin or Ciprofloxacin may be used; however the cautions given above regarding tendon damage apply.

Candida

While by definition more of a side effect than a co-infection, Candida overgrowth seems to be a common feature in tick-borne illness. Candida albicans is yeast that is naturally and normally found in the intestinal tract. In antibiotic therapy where both the "bad" flora and the "good" flora are indiscriminately killed, overgrowth of yeast can occur. This will be discussed in more detail in the next section on naturopathic treatments for tick-borne illness, but there are two primary medications that warrant discussion here.

Nystatin:

Nystatin is an anti-fungal medicine that targets intestinal yeast but is not absorbed through the gut into the blood stream. For this reason, it is a very safe and non-toxic medication as it does not put any stress on the liver. It is taken orally, goes on to kill yeast in the intestinal tract and is excreted through the bowels.

Nystatin is a valuable preventive medication and can be taken along with any antibiotic regimen. It needs to be dosed continuously, with a common dosage of 500,000 units given three times daily, since it does not build up in the system. Especially for women with a tendency towards vaginal yeast infections, Nystatin is recommended concurrently with antibiotic treatment protocols. Nystatin can be used to treat intestinal yeast overgrowth once it has arisen, although it is of limited benefit in more systemic manifestations.

Fluconazole:

Fluconazole (brand name Diflucan) is the heavier hitter of the anti-fungal medications. It does absorb systemically, which makes it more effective for systemic symptoms such as brain fog, vaginal yeast infections, and itchy skin rashes related to yeast overgrowth. On the other hand, the systemic absorption does make it more toxic, and it can add to liver stress when given alongside other medications. Whether used alone or with other drugs, liver tests should be administered periodically while using fluconazole.

If systemic yeast is suspected, one option is to take a 30-day course of fluconazole before long-term antibiotics are commenced, switching then to Nystatin along with antibiotics. Other patients take fluconazole just two to three days per week.

14. GENERAL CONSIDERATIONS FOR TREATMENT AND SAMPLE PROTOCOLS

Intravenous Versus Oral Administration of Antibiotics

Intravenous (IV) administration of antibiotics is another route that can be used in Lyme treatment. Access to IV antibiotics for Lyme can be limited for many, but hopefully, with increased education of the medical community, this situation will change and IV antibiotics will be accessible to a larger cohort.

IV therapy may be indicated in the following conditions:

- Illness duration longer than one year.
- Major neurological involvement.
- Lack of response to oral and/ or intramuscular medications.
- Gastrointestinal function compromise to the point where oral medications are either not getting properly absorbed or are causing excessive GI side effects.

Some of the benefits of IV therapy include:

- Medications can be given in higher doses than oral to achieve higher blood levels.
- Medications given via IV bypass the gastrointestinal tract therefore have fewer GI side effects.
- Most of the medications given orally can be given via IV including doxycycline, azithromycin and metronidazole.

IV antibiotics are not necessarily the easy road or the magic bullet, however. Here are some of the potential issues:

- Having a PICC line or a central line can be very disruptive to activities of daily living. It requires daily maintenance, and risks of infection are always present.
- IV therapy may continue over several months, not just a few weeks. The minimum duration recommended for chronic Lyme is 14 weeks, however if the patient is showing improvement but is still symptomatic, even longer times may be required.
- IV ceftriaxone does not cover all phases of Borrelia nor does it address co-infections, so oral/ IM medications must still be administered for those. Very few patients do all of their three or four mediations via IV.
- IV ceftriaxone can cause biliary sludging and put the individual at risk of having to have their gall bladder surgically removed. (Interestingly, Dr. Burrascano believes that the gall bladder might be a reservoir of infection and has observed that his patients who do not have a gall bladder fare slightly better overall). Any surgery can be stressful for a Lyme patient, as it involves chemicals, anesthesia, heightened risk of infection, adrenal and immune stress, and should be avoided where possible.
- IV ceftriaxone still clears through the liver and may still cause imbalances in the intestinal flora. Preventive measures to keep gut flora balanced must be undertaken.

If IV antibiotics are not available or not indicated, a good alternative is intramuscular administration of Bicillin LA. This is a very effective medication, has good central nervous system penetration, and relieves some of the burden on the gastrointestinal system. While still only addressing the spirochete form of Borrelia, and is therefore not a stand-alone therapy, Bicillin LA is one of the most effective antibiotics available for use in patients who do not have penicillin allergies.

Cautions with all antibiotic therapy

Long-term antibiotic therapy does have some potential side effects. Many possible issues can be easily detected with simple blood work done on a regular basis and sensible prophylactic measures.

Liver and kidney function must be checked every month. Multiple antibiotics for long durations can elevate liver enzymes and put stress on the kidneys. Labs include a complete blood count and a comprehensive metabolic panel that includes BUN, creatinine, AST, ALT and GGTP. If liver enzymes become elevated or kidney function is affected, medications may have to be slowed down, doses lowered or ceased for a duration of time until levels normalize.

Some oral antibiotics cause gastrointestinal side effects and imbalances in gut flora. If diarrhea occurs, it may be a sign of yeast (Candida) overgrowth. Severe, ongoing diarrhea should be evaluated for C. difficile (both toxins A and B) as a cause of colitis. Any antibiotics can predispose a person to C. difficile, but ceftriaxone and clindamycin may create a higher risk.

Medications such as telithromycin can prolong the QT interval and interfere with heart rhythm, so patients on this medication should have cardiac monitoring.

Women (and men!) also need to know that antibiotic therapy, especially the tetracycline family, may reduce the effectiveness of the oral contraceptive pill. Alternative birth control should be used while on antibiotic therapy.

While there are some risks to long-term antibiotic use, many of them can be prevented with naturopathic support such as herbs and probiotics. This will be discussed in the next section. In general terms the benefits of long-term therapy usually outweigh the possible risks, and with careful monitoring, there can be minimal impact on the body from long-term treatment.

Antibiotic Therapy During Pregnancy and Breastfeeding

According to Dr. Joseph Burrascano and Dr. Charles Ray Jones, the optimal medications in pregnancy are:

> Amoxicillin - 1 gram four times daily.
> Bicillin LA - 1 injection three times weekly.
> Cefuroxime - 1 gram every 12 hours.
> Azithromycin - 500mg daily.

Starting in the early 80s, the Lyme Disease Foundation in Hartford, Connecticut kept a pregnancy registry over an eleven-year period. They found that women who took adequate amounts of antibiotics during pregnancy showed a very low, in fact almost zero, transmission rate to their baby. Doctors Burrascano and Jones have found similar statistics in their private practices.

At the ILADS annual conference in 2011, pediatric Lyme specialist Charles Ray Jones cited the following figures:

- Women with active Lyme disease who do not take antibiotics have a 50% chance of passing the infection to their child.
- Women who take one antibiotic during pregnancy have a 25% chance of passing Lyme disease to their child.
- Women who take two antibiotics during pregnancy have less than a 5% chance of passing Lyme disease on to their child.

Obviously, many women are reluctant to take antibiotics during pregnancy for fear of harming their baby. Certainly, there are specific medications that are **not** appropriate, such as the tetracycline class of antibiotics, and metronidazole and tinidazole. The medications cited in the prior paragraph are deemed safe in pregnancy. Still, it is a very personal and difficult decision to make. In my opinion, although taking antibiotics during pregnancy is not ideal, it is a far better choice than risking the transmission of Lyme disease to a baby, which could then impact his or her entire life. Since Borrelia spirochetes have been detected in breast milk by PCR testing, the antibiotic regimens above should be continued during this time also, or breast-feeding avoided.

Antibiotic Therapy for Children

Children can be treated with antibiotic therapy, but the medication choices and dosages will be adjusted for them. Tetracyclines are not used in children eight years and younger because of their ability to cause a permanent discoloration of the teeth.

Antibiotics considered safe and effective for children include:

> Amoxicillin - 50mg/ kg/ day divided into doses every 8 hours
> Cefuroxime axetil - 125mg-500mg every 12 hours based
> on weight.
> Azithromycin - 250-500mg daily depending on their weight
> Tinidazole -125-250mg daily depending on their weight.
> May be pulsed two days per week.
> Grapefruit seed extract - may be a better option for covering
> cyst forms in children.

Practical Application

To summarize, the general principles of antibiotic prescribing in chronic Lyme disease are:

- Start with one medication at a time and assess reactions, side effects, Herx reactions and benefits. More resilient patients may add a new medication after two weeks; more sensitive ones may need 4-6 weeks.
- Layer in medications for all three forms of Borrelia.
- Prioritize co-infection treatment based on symptom picture as well as lab results—decipher which co-infection is dominant. If evidence or suspicion of Babesia consider treating that early along with Borrelia.
- Base the aggressiveness of a person's treatment on Herx levels and patient sensitivity.
- Recognize that Lyme disease requires higher doses of medications and for longer durations than typically used. Two years of treatment is not unusual.
- Treat for two months beyond resolution of symptoms.

Following is a summary of medications to consider along with dosing information and some sample protocols. For convenience this information is reprinted in Appendix C.

Medication Summary

Form of Borrelia	Medication Class	Commonly Used Examples
Spirochetes	Penicillins	Amoxicillin, Bicillin LA
	Cephalosporins	Cefuroxime, Ceftriaxone, Cefdinir
Cell-wall deficient	Macrolides	Azithromycin, Clarithromycin
	Tetracyclines	Doxycycline, Minocycline
Cyst forms		Tinidazole, Metronidazole Hydroxychloroquine (Plaquenil), Alinia

The ultimate goal of therapy for Borrelia:

- 1 cell-wall active medication (for spirochetes)
- 2 intracellular medications (for cell-wall deficient forms)
- 1 cyst form medication (for cysts)

Plus medications added for relevant co-infections.

Common Dosages

Penicillins:

• Amoxicillin	1000mg	3-6 daily
• Augmentin XR	2000mg	2x daily
• Bicillin LA	1.2 mill	1 vial injected IM 3x weekly

Cephalosporins:

- Cefuroxime 500mg 3x daily
- Ceftriaxone 2 gram 2 grams twice daily IV 4days/week
- Cefdinir 300mg 2x daily

Macrolides:

- Azithromycin 500mg 1x daily
- Clarithromycin 500mg 2x daily
- Telithromycin 800mg 1x daily

Tetracyclines:

- Minocycline 100mg 3-4x daily
- Doxycycline 100mg 2 twice daily
- Tetracycline 500mg 3-4x daily

Cyst Form medications:

- Metronidazole 500mg 2x daily; 2 weeks on/ 2 weeks off
- Tinidazole 500mg 2x daily; 2 weeks on/ 2 weeks off
- Plaquenil 200mg 2x daily

Babesia medications:

- Mepron 750mg/ 5mL 1-2 teaspoons twice daily
- Malarone 250/ 100mg 2 twice daily
- Lariam 250mg 1 every five days
- Alinia 500mg 2x daily

Bartonella, Ehrlichia, Anaplasma, Rickettsia medications:

- Rifampin 300mg 2x daily
- Levaquin 500mg 1x daily
- Bactrim DS 800/160mg 2x daily

Sample Medication Protocols

Borrelia:
- Doxycycline 200mg twice daily
- After two weeks add Tinidazole 500mg twice daily 2 weeks on/ 2 weeks off
- One month later add Bicillin LA 1.2 million units 3x weekly
- One month later add Clarithromycin 500mg twice daily

Borrelia in a highly sensitive patient:
- Azithromycin 250mg given Monday-Wednesday-Friday
- Add Plaquenil 200mg twice daily
- Build up azithromycin dose until tolerating 500mg daily
- Add oral amoxicillin 1 gram three times daily
- Add minocycline 100mg twice daily

Borrelia in a patient with a penicillin allergy:
- Doxycycline 200mg twice daily
- Cefuroxime 500mg three times daily
- Tinidazole 500mg twice daily, 2 weeks on/ 2 weeks off

Babesia as the dominant infection:
- Plaquenil 200mg twice daily
- Clarithromycin 500mg twice daily
- Mepron 750mg/ 5mL—1 teaspoon twice daily
- After 6-8 weeks—add Mefloquine 250mg every five days
- After 12-14 weeks—add Bactrim DS twice daily

Borrelia + Babesia:
- Doxycycline 400mg daily
- Plaquenil 200mg twice daily
- Azithromycin 500mg daily
- Mepron 5mL twice daily
- Bicillin LA 1.2 mill units 3 times weekly

Borrelia + Bartonella:

- Doxycycline 200mg twice daily
- Tinidazole 500mg twice daily, 2 weeks on/ 2 weeks off
- Rifampin 300mg twice daily
- Bicillin LA 1.2 mill units 3 times weekly, or Cefuroxime 500mg three times daily
- Can add Bactrim DS twice daily

15. FUNDAMENTALS OF NATURAL MEDICINE IN LYME DISEASE

NATURAL MEDICINE PLAYS SUCH A SIGNIFICANT ROLE IN THE treatment of Lyme disease. In fact, I do not believe in using antibiotic protocols without also using supportive natural therapies alongside them—that is where side effects and unwanted effects on the body occur. Some people decide not to do antibiotic therapy at all and rely solely on natural treatments, while others turn to natural treatments as they either cannot tolerate antibiotics or have seen limited benefit from them. As a practitioner I will only treat Lyme disease with antibiotics in conjunction with the profound benefit and protection of naturopathic support. In my opinion, a combination of both is the preferred approach.

Natural medicines and therapeutics do everything from supporting detoxification and offsetting Herx reactions to actually killing bugs, balancing hormones and supporting immune function.

Different kinds of naturopathic modalities include nutrition, herbal medicine, homeopathy, manual therapies such as massage therapy and cranio-sacral therapy, detoxification therapies, chelation agents (for heavy metal detox), frequency-based therapies such as Rife therapy, salt/ C protocol, enzyme therapies and the list goes on. There are literally hundreds of modalities that can be implemented.

In my practice, I rely heavily on herbal medicines, the use of specific nutrient combinations, and dietary modifications to support and enhance Lyme disease treatment.

The Role of Natural Therapies with Antibiotic Protocols

Naturopathic therapies are primarily used with antibiotics to prevent or offset any possible side effects. The three main aspects to be addressed are:

- Supporting detoxification to minimize Herxheimer reactions
- Preventing liver and kidney stress during antibiotic therapy
- Keeping gut flora balanced and preventing yeast overgrowth

1. Supporting detoxification to minimize Herxheimer reactions

We have already discussed how Herxheimer reactions can occur when antimicrobial therapy is undertaken, whether natural or pharmaceutical. Herx reactions involve a worsening of a person's current or typical symptoms, caused by the release of endotoxins when bacteria, yeast or parasites are killed off, and caused by inflammatory processes as the immune system is engaged to target the exposed infections.

If a Herx gets too severe, antibiotics may need to be reduced or even stopped while the body catches up and clears the toxins. Many people with Lyme have somewhat limited detoxification capacity anyway, and so Herx reactions can become a major issue. Herxes can also be dangerous to the patient, especially when vital functions such as heart function and breathing or swallowing are affected. And of course, Herxes simply make people feel terrible—they can intensify symptoms of pain, inflammation, joint swelling or stiffness, cognitive problems, sleep disturbance, debilitating fatigue and so on. Lyme disease never feels great, so the concept of it getting worse with treatment can be daunting for many, especially when it can last for days to weeks.

In many ways, one's success in recovering from Lyme disease is closely related to one's ability to detoxify, and Herxheimer reactions can be the limiting factor in the progression of treatment if these mechanisms are compromised. Thankfully, naturopathic treatments can greatly improve this by facilitating detoxification in the body. *I prefer detoxification support to be given in advance of any antibiotic therapy to prepare the body.* The body's detox systems should be upregulated before the neurotoxins

are kicked up—trying to get control of it mid-way thr
difficult task.

There are a few remedies that I use to minimize Herxhe
and they work synergistically together.

The first is an herb called Smilax, or Chinese Sarsaparilla.
neutralizing neurotoxins so it is a first-line choice in Herx reac ..is. In
a very few patients, it can cause a slight detox reaction itself, but only in
the most sensitive few. For most, it provides relief from Herxing, and is
considered a gentle herb that is neuro-protective.

It also has anti-inflammatory properties so it can help joint and muscle
pain. I have had patients who were able to reduce or eliminate pain
medications with the introduction of Smilax due to both its detox and
anti-inflammatory properties.

It is important to use Smilax glabrae (as opposed to other kinds of Smilax)
as it crosses the blood-brain barrier. This gives it an edge in neurological
Lyme, where it can help with cognitive symptoms such as brain fog and
memory issues, numbness/ tingling, nerve pain and other neurological
deficits.

Glutathione is my next favorite remedy for supporting detoxification
and minimizing the impact of Herx reactions. Glutathione, which protects every cell against oxidative stress and damage, is one of the key
antioxidants in the body. It helps other antioxidants in the cells remain
in their active form and also plays a role in DNA synthesis and repair,
enhancement of the immune system, and prevention of fat oxidation.
Glutathione is a key element in liver detoxification and is liver protective.

I find that glutathione tends to improve cognitive issues in patients, which
is usually most welcome. Interestingly, studies have shown glutathione
levels to be lower in patients with Parkinson's disease. While we do not
have copious research data to demonstrate this, it is a logical prediction
that many Lyme patients have reduced glutathione levels also.

tathione must be taken in a specific form. If simply taken as a generic glutathione capsule, it will not be highly usable and absorbable by the body. More sophisticated delivery systems have been developed, my favorite being the liposomal reduced L-glutathione. The reduced glutathione is superior over the oxidized; do not worry about the biochemistry—one is useful, the other is not. You want the useful one. The liposomal delivery system means that even though it is taken orally, it is absorbed through the mucous membranes of the mouth and digestive tract, rather than being "digested" in the gut (which is where the loss of absorption occurs as it literally is converted into an oxidized form).

Glutathione can also be very effective when given intravenously—higher doses can be administered, and it goes directly into the blood stream. Availability and cost of this route are usually limiting factors. Transdermal (on the skin) glutathione creams and gels are other options and absorb well. I still prefer the oral liposomal form for convenience and effectiveness. As anyone who takes glutathione can attest, it is a sulfur-based compound and that is evident in the taste. Most people do not want to rub that smell into their skin and carry it around on them all day! Researched Nutritionals, the brand I prefer for glutathione, has released an orange-flavored version, which most people prefer.

The other aspect of minimizing Herx reactions is to bind the toxins to facilitate their removal. Smilax and glutathione are great at neutralizing toxins, but we also have to get them out of the body.

Chlorella can be a good binding agent and works well for drawing out heavy metals also. Some people find it upsetting to the gastrointestinal tract. Other good binders include apple pectin, bentonite clay and activated charcoal. Generally speaking, a diet high in fiber will help elimination through the bowels by its sweeping effect. Ground flax seed or psyllium husk integrated into a daily protein smoothie work well. Binders are generally considered to be substances that stay in the digestive tract and absorb toxins that are dumped there via the bile, as most fat-soluble toxins are.

A summary of ideas to manage Herxes is given in Appendix D.

2. Preventing liver and kidney stress during antibiotic therapy

When taking long-term antibiotics and multiple antibiotics, one of the risks is the extra work the liver and kidneys must do to detoxify and eliminate the medications. As a caution, we check liver and kidney function through lab testing at least once a month.

More common than kidney problems is an elevation in liver enzymes, which can be mild or severe. In some cases, medications must be reduced or ceased to allow enzyme levels to come down, which interrupts treatment.

As always, prevention is better than cure. Natural remedies that support liver function should be in place even before any medications are commenced.

Glutathione is definitely one of the key nutrients for the liver as it helps the liver remove chemicals that are foreign to the body. It is no coincidence that in the body, glutathione levels are highest in the liver and kidneys, two of the major organs of elimination. Glutathione also helps with the detoxification of heavy metals, which are often a problem for Lyme patients (more on that later). Its upregulation of liver enzyme systems and its ability to bind toxins in the body including chemical residues of antibiotics and other medications make it a valuable remedy for assisting the liver and kidneys.

There are several herbs that have great liver protective and liver cleansing properties. Dandelion root is one of my favorites because it is safe, gentle, effective and will not interfere with medications. Dandelion leaf can be used too, although it has a greater affinity for the kidneys, restoring mineral balance as it flushes out toxins.

Dandelion root's benefit comes from oils and bitter resins that stimulate digestive function and bile flow, combined with a viscous fiber which binds and transports toxins out of the body. It can be taken as an herbal tincture or as a tea. Dandelion root tea makes a great coffee substitute and is actually better for the liver than coffee, which just adds to the toxic burden!

Milk thistle is perhaps the best-known liver herb. It has been used exten-sively to protect liver cells against toxins and the toxic effects of medica-tions. It contains flavonoids, which prevent liver cells from damage and also aid in their regeneration. The only drawback of milk thistle is that is does not combine well with Mepron and Malarone. It can interfere with their absorption, so people taking these two Babesia medications should not take milk thistle.

RestorMedicine Detox Support Formula #1 is a liver formula that con-tains milk thistle and is used in patients not on Mepron or Malarone; Detox Support Formula #2 has the milk thistle removed so that is a good choice for those on Mepron or Malarone.

Licorice root is another herb that has great benefit for the liver. Studies have shown that licorice can increase the body's production of inter-feron, which supports both liver function and immune function. Its anti-inflammatory effects reduce medication-related liver inflammation and at the same time provide antioxidants to protect liver cells.

3. Keeping gut flora balanced and preventing yeast overgrowth

Antibiotics can disrupt the gut flora. In the intestinal tract there are billions of naturally occurring yeast and bacteria. The gut contains an entire ecosystem, which maintains a delicate balance. This ecosystem functions to maximize assimilation of nutrients and provides a complex immune system of its own. The gut has a complex system of defense in place given that the gut is one of the first-line points of entry into the body and consequently is exposed to so many outside influences.

Antibiotics may be good for eradicating bacteria in the body, which we want in bacterial illnesses such as Lyme disease. However they are not discriminating. They will also have an effect against the healthy bacteria in the gut. If the healthy bacteria in the gut are reduced, opportunis-tic yeast such as Candida can gain a foothold and grow beyond their normal healthy levels. Candida albicans and other strains of yeast are completely natural and normal in the gut; it is when they overgrow that problems arise.

Yeast overgrowth may appear as intestinal gas and bloating, a white coating on the tongue, vaginal irritation and infections for women, itchy skin rashes, increased brain fog and fatigue, among other things.

You will not be surprised to hear me say that here, prevention is the key. High potency, high quality probiotic supplements must be used along with antibiotics to help keep the gut flora in balance and prevent yeast overgrowth. Optimally, a variety of different strains of acidophilus and bifido bacteria will be used, and many good probiotics provide that. There is a type of yeast called Saccharomyces boulardii that is actually supplemented to prevent yeast also. It is counterintuitive to give a yeast to prevent yeast, but the goal is simply to supply enough of the "good yeast" that the "bad yeast" cannot get a foothold.

Most probiotics contain living organisms and therefore must be refrigerated to maintain their potency. The exception to this is soil-based probiotics (such as Prescript-Assist by Researched Nutritionals). Soil-based probiotics work slightly differently and are less susceptible to heat. They can be a good option while traveling or when refrigerated probiotics are not practical.

Probiotics must be taken at least two hours apart from antibiotics, otherwise the antibiotics can kill them off, too. This is true of prescription antibiotics, but it also applies to any natural remedy that has antimicrobial properties (such as teasel root, samento, olive leaf and grapefruit seed extract), as well as anti-fungal medications and herbs. I suggest taking probiotics at night before bed so that they have several hours to colonize in the gut before an assault by another dose of antibiotics. At least 100 billion live organisms per day must be taken as a prevention/ maintenance dose; for people with yeast issues 200 billion live organisms per day are needed. The RestorProbiotic Powder contains 200 billion live organisms per scoop and has helped many patients maintain healthy digestive function.

Natural medicine can be very helpful in anti-fungal therapy if yeast overgrowth does arise and we will cover than in the next section. For now, the important thing is to recognize the importance of probiotics in the prevention of gut flora imbalances during antibiotic therapy.

General Naturopathic Principles

Everything discussed above, while being crucial when taking antibiotics, is just as applicable for those not on antibiotics. Supporting detoxification is imperative for all chronic Lyme patients. Aside from the infection itself, most chronically ill patients have some component of toxicity contributing to their illness. This can worsen muscle and joint pain, brain fog, fatigue and neurological deficits.

More on Detoxification

Part of toxin build up may come from defects in the methylation pathway. The methylation pathway is responsible for a host of different metabolic functions, including detox, energy production and certain brain chemicals such as serotonin. If methylation pathways are not supported, then these functions will be compromised. Methylation, as the name suggests, requires "methyl groups" to feed it. Certain natural supplements can act as "methyl donors," feeding the raw materials to fuel the pathway, just like putting petrol in a car.

Supplements that support methylation include dimethylglycine (DMG), trimethylglycine (TMG) and methylcobalamin (a form of the vitamin B12). Methyl-B12 given by injection three times weekly can provide a great boost to energy and immune function, while supporting methylation pathways for detoxification. If injections are not available, sublingual forms of MB12 are the next best. Folic acid is also an important nutrient for methylation, and is best given in the form of 5-methyl-tetrahydrafolate.

MTHFR genetic markers can be tested to assess for defects in methylation and can help guide the appropriate supplementation.

Part of supporting detoxification is aiming for a more alkaline state. Nutritional principles for this will be covered in the next section. Supplementing with chlorophyll or chlorella can help. I encourage patients to drink a glass of warm water with the juice of one lemon squeezed in it on a daily basis. This can be especially helpful during Herxes as it seems to reduce the intensity of symptoms.

Other easy at-home remedies to support detox include taking baths with either Epsom salts or baking soda. Epsom salts are magnesium sulfate. The magnesium is very relaxing to the muscles, easing aches and pains, while also promoting relaxation and sleep; the sulfate part promotes detoxification. Baking soda is used more for its alkaline effects, not as much to help detox.

Castor oil packs are an age-old remedy but still have benefit. When placed over the liver, castor oil packs have been known to stimulate gall bladder function and bile flow, and clear stagnation and toxic build up in the liver. If liver enzymes become elevated during antibiotic therapy, castor oil packs are a good addition to the program to help reduce them. They can be done daily during these times, but generally 3-4 times weekly is sufficient. I have also found castor oil packs to be useful when used on specific areas of pain and inflammation. Instructions as to how to use castor oil packs are given in Appendix E.

As previously mentioned, while the liver is responsible for detoxifying chemicals, hormones and metabolites of our foods, it is not the only organ of elimination. Once the liver converts harmful toxins into non-harmful metabolites, they are excreted through the skin, lungs, bowels and kidneys. Subsequently anything that can be done to support these organs can be helpful. An example is far-infrared (FIR) sauna. FIR sauna operates at lower temperatures than regular saunas, but being a different type of heat wave it actually penetrates the tissues more deeply assisting the cells in releasing toxins and clearing them through the skin. FIR sauna is especially good for heavy metal detox, which will be discussed later in this section, as it helps release toxins from fat cells.

Helping to flush the kidneys by drinking two liters of water a day is beneficial. For the lungs, either sauna therapy or some aerobic exercise stimulates their function. The bowels are a major channel of elimination. It is crucial to have at least one, preferably two, bowel movements per day. Ground flax or psyllium husk can be added to smoothies or food; extra magnesium or vitamin C promotes bowel motility (too much will give diarrhea however); and some will need to supplement with soluble and insoluble fibers such as apple pectin, guar gum and aloe.

Binding agents are generally not absorbed from the intestinal tract and can help remove toxins by holding on to them and "escorting" them out of the body, after the toxins are dumped into the gut via bile (bile is one of the major routes of elimination for many toxins, but since 90% of bile is reabsorbed, it is important to take binding agents so that toxins do not get reabsorbed by the body). Activated charcoal is a good binder—it has a lattice structure that can trap toxins—and for this reason is often given in cases of accidental poisoning. Taken two to three hours after an antimicrobial that is creating die-off can ease Herx-type symptoms. Chlorella is often used in heavy metal detox as a binder especially in the gut. Chlorella alone will not be sufficient to mobilize heavy metals from the tissues, but can be taken alongside chelation protocols and also may be a good idea to take when eating a meal containing seafood, which may possibly be contaminated with heavy metals such as mercury. In cases of severe neurotoxicity during Herx reactions, a medication called Cholestyramine is sometimes used. It is a prescription medication that it used to lower cholesterol (again, by binding the fatty acids in bile), but has been used in some cases of chronic infectious illness and particularly where mold toxicity may be a factor. Again, binding to the bile to prevent reabsorption is one of the keys to eliminating toxins from the body.

The other detoxification channel that is often forgotten is the lymphatic system. The lymphatic system is like the storm drains of the body—it filters the blood and removes toxic debris, bringing it back through a series of vessels towards the heart where it can be dumped into the larger blood vessels to be taken to the liver. Essentially, it keeps the toxic muck from clogging up the blood vessels, and can also function to deliver foreign invaders such as viruses and bacteria to the immune system. Lymphatic flow can be supported using herbs such as cleavers, burdock and pokeroot. Dry skin brushing can also be an easy way to gently enhance lymphatic drainage (see Appendix F for detailed information on how to do skin brushing). Lymphatic drainage massage is a specific massage technique that accelerates lymph flow; however it can also release a flood of toxins and make people feel temporarily worse afterwards. Exercise will also help keep the lymphatic system moving, especially jumping on a rebounder.

Inflammation

Inflammation is a major part of chronic infectious illness such as Lyme disease. Inflammation also arises from Herxheimer reactions, which increases immune chemicals called cytokines. Inflammation causes much of the pain and swelling in the joints, muscles and other connective tissue in Lyme disease. It can also cause swelling around the lining of the heart, and in the brain.

Managing inflammation is an important aspect of Lyme treatment, and natural remedies can certainly support this. The dietary influences on inflammation will be discussed in the next section on nutrition. I use herbs extensively to reduce inflammation. One of the main ones is white willow. It is used to make aspirin and is the plant from which salicylic acid is derived.

Another effective anti-inflammatory agent is turmeric. Often as effective as pharmaceutical anti-inflammatories but without the side effects, turmeric can be a potent pain reliever through its inhibition of Cox-2 pathways. It has the added benefit of being a great liver detoxifier.

Another approach to reducing inflammation is to use proteolytic enzymes. Whereas digestive enzymes are taken with food to help break the food down into easily absorbable molecules, proteolytic enzymes are taken away from food and are intended to be absorbed systemically and break down the by-products of the inflammatory process. They can help reduce the signs and symptoms of inflammation, which are heat, redness and pain. Used extensively in musculoskeletal inflammation, proteolytic enzymes can have a much broader impact by facilitating healthy immune response and preventing auto-immunity that may occur when the body is in a chronic inflammatory state.

Certain healthy fats can be taken to reduce inflammation. While the "good fats" are omega-3, omega-6 and omega-9s, the omega-3 fats have the most potent anti-inflammatory effects and they should be supplemented. We will discuss this more in the next section on nutritional strategies for Lyme disease. Fish and flax oil can both be supplemented at doses of two to six grams per day to provide omega-3 fatty acids and to help dampen inflammation.

Immune Function

Immune support is a crucial part of Lyme disease treatment. Our immune systems are our body's defense systems. They help to fight the infection, regulate inflammation and provide protection against other foreign invaders such as other viruses and bacteria.

In medicine we use the term "host defenses," which refers to the immune system of the person with the disease (the host). Largely, ones immune system regulates ones ability to fight disease. Lyme patients need to support their immune function so that their body can contribute to the cause by killing off some of the infection through natural mechanisms. The stronger the immune system, the greater the ability to overcome and eradicate infection. While we do not want an overactive immune response, which can lead to auto-immunity, we do want a well-balanced and highly regulated immune system with sufficient power to fight infection.

Unfortunately, Lyme disease and related co-infections can dampen immune function. The co-infection Ehrlichia is particularly renowned for lowering the white blood cell count (white blood cells are immune cells); Borrelia can have the same effect. As previously discussed this is one of the reasons that lab testing for Lyme disease is so challenging—the immune reaction needed to register a positive result is lessened by the infection itself.

To boost immune function, we have a variety of natural options. Since the immune system has different components—B cells (antibodies), T cells and natural killer (NK) cells—it is preferred to choose a variety of immune agents to support all aspects.

Transfer factors are small protein molecules that serve as messengers for the immune system, allowing for a faster and more efficient immune response. They train your immune system to function optimally and respond better to invaders. What is amazing about transfer factors is that they can be targeted for specific infections. A Lyme-specific transfer factor can actually help the immune system to identify Borrelia and go into attack mode on that specific infection. A combination of general transfer factors and targeted transfer factors is ideal for the highest level of immune support.

Transfer factors also support Natural Killer (NK) cell activity. NK cells are the Pac-Men of the immune system running around after the foreign invaders (bacteria, yeast, parasites etc). They are also designed to kill cancer cells. If you recall we discussed the CD-57 as being a marker on the NK cell—this can be quantitatively measured to assess how burdened the immune system is with Lyme disease. NK cells are a vital part of immune defense.

Beta glucans are also immune-fortifying molecules. They are sugars that are found in the cell walls of bacteria, fungi, yeasts, algae and some plants such as oats and barley. The beta glucans found in most supplements are extracted from the cell walls of the yeast Saccromyces cerevisaie (the final product is an extract only and does not contain yeast). Once extracted, they function to enhance recognition of invaders, and they bind with macrophages, a type of immune cell, to set off a cascade of heightened cellular response.

Colostrum is a high-protein substance that is found in the milk of mammals. Colostrum contains immune and growth factors including antibodies such as IgG, IgE, IgA, IgM and IgD (we talked about IgM and IgG antibodies in relation to laboratory testing). Colostrum is considered a natural source of such immune cells. In fact, the purpose of colostrum in mammal's milk is to confer immunity to the offspring while their own immune system is still developing. Colostrum is extracted from the milk so only very scant traces of lactose and milk proteins are left behind. Those avoiding dairy can still safely take colostrum.

Medicinal mushrooms such as reishi, shitake and maitake have been used for centuries in traditional Chinese medicine, and evidence shows the ancient Egyptians also relied on their health benefits. Mushrooms benefit the immune system with their naturally occurring beta glucans, but they also contain other polysaccharides that upregulate the immune system and provide antimicrobial activity. Mushrooms may also have hormone-modulating properties. Some people with extreme Candida and yeast overgrowth, or with sensitivity to fungi, may not do well with medicinal mushrooms; however for many, they are a great addition to an immune protocol.

Herbs that support immune function are a helpful addition too. While some herbalists do not support its use in chronic health issues, astragalus is an herb that I use with good results. Along with its immune benefits, it also has mild antibacterial and anti-inflammatory activity.

While healthy levels of all vitamins and minerals are necessary for healthy immune function, vitamins C and D are particularly important.

Vitamin C boosts the immune system through its influence on the production and function of white blood cells and antibodies, and it enhances interferon, which coats the cell surfaces to help ward off infection. It is also a powerful antioxidant, and in that role it protects immune cells from being damaged by toxins in the body.

Vitamin D has received much attention in recent years. It is associated with reducing inflammation and can have pain-modulating benefits. It also functions both as a fat-soluble vitamin within the body and also as a hormone, and has known benefit to the immune system. Adequate levels of vitamin D are necessary for the signaling and activation of T cells (one of the branches of the immune system) when a foreign invader is detected. When the immune cell is presented with a pathogen, it will put out a receptor for vitamin D, and once bound, that complex will signal T cells to mobilize, producing either NK cells to kill off the pathogen, or T-helper cells that train the immune system to remember that threat, allowing it to be more efficient next time it encounters it. Studies have found that a deficiency of vitamin D will hinder this process and reduce immune response.

Given that a strong immune system is a key component in being able to fight infection, moderate inflammation and recover from Lyme disease, it seems only sensible to utilize some of the powerful tools nature has given us.

Natural Antibiotics and Antimicrobials

Some people opt not to take pharmaceutical antibiotics, some are restricted by drug allergies or medication side effects, and some feel that they need extra antimicrobial help along with their antibiotics. I have seen natural antimicrobial agents work effectively against Lyme disease, its co-infections and some of the other commonly found pathogens in chronic illness such as yeast and viruses. When starting any antimicrobial therapy, I like to start out with herbs instead of antibiotics. It is easier to gauge sensitivity levels and a person's tendency to Herx with plant-based medicines that have fewer side effects than antibiotics.

Please note that the below information is just a sampling of available non-pharmaceutical treatments for these infections. Literally dozens of other options exist, and the below information is intended as an introduction, not a comprehensive guide.

Borrelia

Samento—perhaps one of the best-known herbs for Borrelia, samento (also known as Cats Claw and Prima Una de Gato) has been used widely as a stand-alone therapy and in conjunction with antibiotics. The plant contains constituents known as quinovic acid glycosides, which are natural precursors to quinolones, a class of pharmaceutical antibiotics (of which Levaquin is one).

Teasel root—possibly my favorite herb for Borrelia, teasel root is highly effective while still being gentle on the body. It is a potent antimicrobial and also has some anti-inflammatory properties. Drop doses (up to 10-15 daily) are typically all that is required. Teasel can provoke significant Herx reactions at the start of treatment.

Guaicum—this herb gained popularity in the sixteenth century as a cure for syphilis. Although it is not widely used in the United States, it is still used in Europe for spirochetal illnesses, of which Lyme disease and syphilis are categorized. Guaiacum also has anti-inflammatory properties and as such is used for arthritic and rheumatological manifestations of Lyme.

Grapefruit seed extract (GSE)—not to be confused with grapeseed extract (which is an antioxidant), grapefruit seed extract can be given to address the cyst forms of Borrelia. While human studies are not available, grapefruit seed extract did appear to eradicate Borrelia cysts in vitro (in the test tube). While perhaps not as potent as the medications for cyst forms, grapefruit seed extract is definitely a good option when medications are not tolerated or not available. (Samento and Banderol are options for cyst forms and biofilm too).

Babesia

Artemisinin - this is the active ingredient from the plant Artemesia annua, an anti-malarial, anti-parasitic herb (also known as Sweet Wormwood). It is effective against the co-infection Babesia, which is an intracellular parasite that creates an illness similar to malaria. Some practitioners give high doses of artemisinin (up to 500mg three times daily) but the Herx reaction can be profound. Lower doses of 200-400mg per day are more manageable. Because of its potential to create liver stress, it is advised to take one week off per month from dosing and check liver enzymes periodically.

Cryptolepis - with less of a track record, Cryptolepis has still been used more recently for Babesiosis with seemingly good results. Accessibility and supply can be an issue; it is made from plants grown in Africa and can be challenging to source.

Enula - this product is made by NutraMedix, and is a combination of three different herbs—Elecampane, Jalapa and Blood Wiss. It is used in the treatment of Babesia, as well as parasitic worms. Also as an antimicrobial it has been shown to be effective in the treatment of MRSA.

Byron White's A-BAB formula is another effective option and can be used in conjunction with artemisinin.

Bartonella

Houttuynia is an herb used by QingCai Zhang, author of *Lyme Disease and Modern Chinese Medicine*. His product is called HH2 and is highly effective against Bartonella. This is the primary natural remedy I use for Bartonella.

The Nutramedix herbs developed by Dr Cowden including Cumanda and Banderol, and the newer Byron White A-Bart formula, have also been used to treat Bartonella. Stephen Buhner recommends the herb Sida acuta stating that it protects the red blood cells against invasion by the Bartonella organisms.

Candida/ Yeast

There are many effective anti-fungals found in nature. The following are just a sampling, but I have found them to be effective. Anti-fungals seem to produce the best results when rotated—some people switch them every week, others every month. I tend to use combinations of anti-fungals at the same time for maximum coverage.

Grapefruit seed extract - already mentioned for its cyst-busting properties for Borrelia, grapefruit seed extract is also an effective anti-fungal. For this dual benefit it is often used in Lyme treatment. A 1990 study published in the Journal of Orthomolecular Medicine also showed grapefruit seed extract to be effective against molds such as Aspergillus and Penicillium species.[1]

Garlic - one of nature's best anti-fungals, garlic has many other health giving properties. It is antimicrobial against a wide variety of pathogens while concurrently supporting the immune system. It also has a beneficial influence on cholesterol and blood sugar levels. Garlic cloves added to food are an easy and inexpensive way to get garlic, but for more potency, it can also be supplemented in liquid or capsule forms.

Caprylic acid - found in coconut oil, caprylic acid not only kills yeast by interfering with the cell wall of Candida but also restores healthy stomach acidity, allowing for better digestion of foods, especially proteins. Caprylic acid is typically well tolerated.

Oregano oil - oil of oregano is a potent anti-fungal that has been used in Mediterranean regions for many years. The chemical compounds in oregano react with the water in the bloodstream to dehydrate and kill the Candida yeast. It produces less resistance than other anti-fungals so it can be used effectively long term. Gastrointestinal side effects can be an issue, especially with liquid forms, so gel caps are usually better tolerated. Oregano oil also has some activity against Bartonella.

Pau d'Arco - originating from the Amazon basin, Pau d'Arco contains a range of constituents that have yeast-fighting activity. The primary way this herb is taken is as a tea, although it can be taken as a tincture too.

Olive leaf - another herb that supports the immune system while also having potent anti-fungal properties. Olive leaf is also very effective against parasites and viruses, making it a good supplement for chronic Lyme sufferers. High dose olive leaf should not be taken while taking antibiotic therapies, but moderate doses show considerable benefit.

Viruses

While not theoretically co-infections of Lyme, many chronic Lyme patients have chronic viral infections, notably Epstein Barr virus (EBV), Cytomega-lovirus (CMV), Human Herpes Virus 6 (HHV-6), and Herpes Simplex 1 and 2 (HSV 1 & 2). Natural remedies can assist the body in managing these viruses and prevent them from adding to Lyme symptoms.

Olive leaf - already mentioned as an anti-fungal, olive leaf has excellent anti-viral properties. It works by interfering with critical amino acid production essential for viruses, by inactivating viruses or by preventing virus shedding, and by directly penetrating infected cells to stop viral replication in the case of retroviruses.

Lauricidin - this extract is derived from coconut oil. It works by binding to the lipid-protein envelope of the virus, preventing it from attaching to and entering host cells, and therefore preventing it from replicating. Lauricidin is also used as an anti-fungal and anti-bacterial, and has immune strengthening properties. One of the advantages of lauricidin is that it kills off unwanted pathogens without killing off the good flora in the gut.

Biofilm

Biofilm, as we discussed in section two, is the mucopolysaccharide matrix (aka "sticky goo") in which Borrelia hide to evade detection by the immune system and resist antimicrobial treatment. It is probable that biofilm needs to be addressed in every Lyme patient; however, it should definitely be considered in a person who is doing a lot of antimicrobial therapy with very limited improvement. A summary of biofilm protocols is given in Appendix G.

Most of the remedies used to help break down biofilm are enzyme based and blood-thinning agents. Their goal is to break through the sticky substance so that the bacteria can be exposed to antimicrobial agents.

Lumbrokinase is one of the blood-thinning agents used to address biofilm. Its cousin, nattokinase, is also used but has somewhat lesser efficacy (but is also less expensive). Proteolytic enzymes such as those used in anti-inflammatory supplements can be helpful too. Calcium EDTA, while often thought of as a heavy metal chelator, is given along with lumbrokinase to break down the bonds within the biofilm substance. It does this by forming complexes with the ions in the matrix, rendering it less able to hold together. Also, biofilm is known to contain various metals, which may also explain why calcium EDTA is effective here.

Once biofilm is being dissolved, there may be a greater Herx reaction, as more bacteria and parasites are newly exposed and open to being killed off. This, of course, is the goal, but an acceleration of the process should be anticipated and extra detox support given.

Another aspect of the biofilm protocol is to increase fiber intake to ensure that the bowels are getting adequately swept, and that microbial debris and toxins are being eliminated. Finally, adequate probiotics are needed to replace and rebalance healthy microbial flora.

Digestive Health

We have already discussed the need for probiotics to maintain healthy digestion, and some of the natural remedies used to control yeast ɔwth in the gut. However, naturopathic remedies can also be used ιᴏ address other problems in the digestive system.

Gastrointestinal Infections

Infections in the gut can be bacterial or parasitic in nature.

Helicobacter pylori (H. pylori) are bacteria that infect the stomach, causing reflux/ heartburn, burping, stomach pain, and compromised ability to digest food, particularly proteins. The bacteria interfere with the cells in the stomach that produce hydrochloric acid (HCL), which is necessary for the proper digestion of food. H. pylori is often treated with antibiotics. From a natural standpoint, mastic gum is one of the key agents that can eradicate H. pylori. Zinc carnosine is also helpful. Deglycyrrhizinated licorice (DGL) assists by coating and healing the esophageal and stomach tissue that may have become irritated by the infection.

I have observed that sometimes stomach issues are assumed to be a side effect of medications, when really they may be caused by H. pylori. Many people taking proton-pump inhibitors and other antacids could be spared from years of these medications by an accurate diagnosis of H. pylori.

Intestinal parasites are common in chronic Lyme patients, perhaps because of a general lowering of immune function and increased susceptibility to pathogens. Intestinal parasites such as Cryptosporidium parvum, Blastocystis hominis and Entamoeba histolytica can cause symptoms such as gas, bloating, constipation, diarrhea (sometimes alternating between the two) and abdominal pain. Again, long-term antibiotic use can often be the assumed cause of gut issues such as these, but ongoing, evaluation for parasites can be useful.

Herbs that have strong anti-parasitic activity include black walnut, wormwood, gentian, clove and yellow dock. Garlic and olive leaf are used here too.

Side Effects of Antibiotics

Certainly, gastrointestinal side effects, predominantly nausea and diarrhea are among the most common in Lyme treatment.

One of the best remedies for nausea is ginger. Whether it is taken as a tea, added to food, or ingested in dried forms, ginger has a long history of use for nausea, whether caused by medications, pregnancy or motion sickness. I prefer the ginger root cut into small pieces and boiled for 10 to 15 minutes. Stevia (a natural sweetener and sugar alternative) can be added for sweetness.

Peppermint is also good for nausea as well as irritable bowel type symptoms and indigestion. It can be taken as a tea, which is preferred, or drunk with one or two drops of peppermint oil mixed in water.

Some people find that essential oils of peppermint and lavender can help relieve nausea when diffused into the air.

Mild diarrhea caused by medications can often be offset by increased probiotic use, anti-fungal therapies such as those listed earlier in the section, and/ or the gut healing nutrients listed below under "leaky gut." Peppermint tea is also useful. Any ongoing or severe diarrhea should be evaluated for Clostridia difficile, which is a possible result of antibiotic therapy.

I have also seen increased fiber intake help diarrhea (probably due to its binding capabilities)—especially soluble fibers such as apple pectin and chia seeds. Insoluble fibers such as psyllium husk can be too irritating for some. As a binder, activated charcoal can mop up toxins, which reduces diarrhea and also the severity of Herxheimer reactions.

For bowel regularity I suggest a tablespoon of ground flax seeds taken daily, either sprinkled on food or blended into a smoothie. If constipation is an issue, the safest approaches are fibers such as flax or rice bran, or high dose vitamin C or magnesium.

Leaky Gut
Leaky gut refers to the phenomena where the cells in the wall of the small intestine become spaced out beyond what they should be. Ordinarily, the junctions between the cells are only large enough to let single particles of digested food into the blood stream for transport to other parts of the

body. When the junctions open up, larger food particles can get through. This causes an immune reaction, as the immune system is trained to see single particles as "good" and clusters of particles as "bad." Of course, whenever "bad" happens, the immune system rushes to attack, which inherently leads to inflammation that can affect the entire body.

Eating foods that are inflammatory (more about this in the next chapter) or that one has allergies or intolerances to, having yeast imbalances and having unresolved chronic infections in the gut are also precursors to leaky gut.

Of all the nutrients that can be used to repair leaky gut, perhaps the most effective is the amino acid L-glutamine. Glutamine is healing to the intestinal wall, and can calm symptoms fairly rapidly. Slippery elm used as a gruel (powder mixed with water and eaten) is also very effective, as is aloe vera juice. Deglycyrrhizinated licorice can be used for intestinal healing (as well as esophageal healing) in combination with the other nutrients. Marshmallow tea is of great benefit for soothing and healing the gut.

Energy

One of the primary symptoms of chronic Lyme disease is fatigue. To some extent, fatigue will improve as the infection is eradicated, however there are things that may help to improve it along the way.

Three of the major causes of fatigue in chronic illness are adrenal fatigue, mitochondrial insufficiency and methylation defects. Let us explore each in more detail.

Adrenal Fatigue

The adrenals are the stress management centers of the body. Cortisol, one of the hormones they produce, is nicknamed the "stress hormone." When there is a stress on the body—whether an emotional stress, or equally a physical stress such as chronic infection, pain and inflammation—the adrenals respond by increasing cortisol output. This is a healthy mechanism that helps the body to compensate for the stress by giving the body an extra boost to deal with whatever is happening.

The problem lies in the fact that so often the stress becomes chronic, it does not go away. Subsequently the adrenal glands work harder and harder to maintain their cortisol output. Their compensatory mechanisms break down and over time cortisol levels will start to fall. Eventually, adrenal exhaustion ensues, reflected by low cortisol readings on labs and feelings of total physical, mental and emotional exhaustion. Cortisol is a natural anti-inflammatory, so it follows that chronically low cortisol allows for more inflammation, and more pain, in the body.

The first step in evaluating adrenal health is accurate testing. While blood levels can be measured, they will only reflect levels at that one particular time of day. Cortisol has a circadian rhythm, so its levels start high in the morning, and ordinarily fall gradually throughout the day and are lowest at night. Low cortisol at night is essential for the immune system to kick in and do its housekeeping (which it does during the night); and to allow restful sleep.

A saliva test can be a convenient way to get that information and can be done at home. A tube of saliva is collected at 8am, 12 noon, 4pm and 8pm, and then cortisol levels can be charted reflecting their levels throughout the day. It is not uncommon to see cortisol levels slump in the afternoon, in line with the typical afternoon energy crash, or levels elevated at night in those with major sleep issues. Granted, blood levels could be measured too, however it would require four samples during the same day, so that is not as practical.

Adrenal support is an important part of the Lyme treatment protocol. Herbs and glandulars (extracts from animal adrenal glands) can both be used. Some herbs are called adaptogens, which means that they balance function. They will upregulate sluggish adrenals, or tone down overactive adrenals. Basically they normalize function whether it is high or low. This is a great option if levels are unbalanced during the day (high at some times and low at others) as there is minimal risk of creating further imbalance.

Some of the more popular adrenal adaptogens include:

- Panax Ginseng (Korean Ginseng)

- Eleuthrococcus (Siberian Ginseng)
- Ashwaghanda
- Rhodiola

Of these, I think of panax ginseng being more energizing and stimulating (too much for some people) while eleuthrococcus and ashwaghanda are more gentle and balancing. Rhodiola is great for the mental and emotional impact of chronic stress.

Licorice root is another valuable adrenal herb. It can build cortisol levels and is used in adrenal insufficiency for this reason. Over time it can cause slight elevations in blood pressure, and it can be slightly estrogenic, so either of those pre-existing issues may make long-term administration problematic in some individuals.

There is also a product called Isocort that contains plant-based cortisol in very small doses (approximately 2-2.5mg per pellet). In people with very low cortisol levels, supplementing this way can bring quick relief from debilitating fatigue and help the adrenals get back on track.

Balancing low cortisol using plant-derived cortisol is very different to giving immune-suppressive steroid drugs such as prednisone. Prednisone is an immune suppressant and *should never be given to a Lyme disease patient* as it further renders their immune system unable to fight the infection. Even if the prednisone reduces inflammation and reduces symptoms, the long-term effects totally negate the benefit. Low dose plant-derived cortisol gives the body the cortisol it needs for the various roles it plays until such a time that the adrenals can recover and take over healthy production. Cortisol is closely tied with the immune system, so chronically low cortisol output restricts immune response just as boosting cortisol levels too much with prednisone also restricts immune response. It is a delicate balancing act.

Another approach to balancing adrenal hormones is to supplement with the precursors DHEA and pregnenolone. Pregnenolone is nicknamed the "grandmother hormone" because it supplies the material needed to produce a host of other adrenal hormones, including progesterone, cortisol, estrogen and testosterone. DHEA can be used as it is, or converted by the body to estrogen or testosterone.

If cortisol levels are too high—as may be the case in less chronic cases where night time elevations interrupt sleep or the adrenals are still trying to compensate for the stressors—the adaptogenic herbs may also be used to regulate those elevations.

Phosphorylated serine is a nutrient (serine is an amino acid) that has been used to dampen elevated cortisol levels. It is taken several hours before bed for nighttime elevations, and in the morning and afternoon for overall high levels.

Finally, full recovery from adrenal fatigue typically requires a reduction in overall lifestyle stressors, as well as a healthy diet low in inflammatory foods and high in B vitamins, especially pantothenic acid (vitamin B5). Additionally, vitamin C is one of the primary nutrients used by the adrenal glands; liposomal vitamin C can have profound healing effects on the adrenal glands.

Mitochondrial Dysfunction

Another cause of low energy in chronic illness is mitochondrial dysfunction. The mitochondria are the little engines within each of our cells that produce our energy. This energy is called adenosine triphosphate, or ATP. If the little engines are not well oiled and well fuelled, slow downs can occur in the production of the ATP, which reduces the energy available for the body to use.

Certain nutrients have been shown to support mitochondrial function. NADH and CoQ10 are two that feed and support the cycle. Alpha-ketoglutaric acid and L-carnitine are others. It is important to note that patients who are taking Mepron or Malarone for Babesiosis should not supplement with CoQ10 while they are on those medications, as the CoQ10 will interfere with the medications and make them less effective.

The other consideration here is that the membrane of the mitochondria contains its own DNA. Therefore if the membrane integrity is compromised, function will be impaired. NT Factor is well researched to provide phospholipids that can be transported from cell to cell and integrated into the mitochondrial membrane, keeping both structure and function optimal.

Supplementary mitochondrial support can help energy production tremendously. Typically, higher doses of the above nutrients are taken for the first two months to facilitate repair of the membrane and accelerate the biochemical pathways, then more moderate doses can be taken after that.

Methylation Defects

We have already discussed methylation defects as a cause of toxin build-up in the body, but it can also be a contributor to fatigue. In part, it ties into adrenal dysfunction, as methylation pathways can be impaired secondary to adrenal exhaustion.

Supporting methylation with methyl-B12 therapy can provide a generous boost of energy and improved mental outlook. One might think that simply taking the vitamin B12 in any form could do this, as B12 is a vitamin that is associated with energy, and to some extent, that is true. Some patients respond well to the forms of B12 that are not methylation-boosters (eg cyanocobalamin and hydroxocobalamin). However, I have seen clinically that far more patients derive benefit from the methyl-B12 therapy, indicating the methyl groups are equally significant. While beyond the scope of this discussion, biochemical markers can be measured through laboratory testing of the blood (MTHFR genetic markers as well as levels of amino acids methionine and cysteine), that indicate whether a person is an under-methylator or over-methylator. This can guide appropriate supplementation.

Hormone Health

Along with adrenal dysfunction, chronic Lyme patients often develop thyroid issues. There are two factors behind this. First, Lyme and co-infections impact the hypothalamus and the pituitary gland, the master regulators in the brain of hormone function; this is why all the hormones can easily get out of whack. Second, the thyroid is quite susceptible to autoimmune issues, and given that Lyme can trigger autoimmune processes within the body, it follows that the thyroid might be in the path of that. Hashimoto's thyroiditis is an autoimmune thyroid condition that often starts with a phase of hyperthyroidism (high thyroid function) but then moves into a longer phase of hypothyroidism (low thyroid function). Antibodies such as anti-TPO and anti-thyroglobulin antibodies are helpful markers to evaluate this autoimmune component. General testing for TSH, free T3 and free T4 show actual levels of thyroid hormones. Reverse T3 can be helpful as some people convert T4 to reverse T3 instead of the more active form of T3 itself. Even patients in the lower end of the normal ranges may have clinical signs and symptoms of hypothyroidism and would benefit from thyroid support.

Some people need to take thyroid hormone supplements to boost their thyroid function. The optimal way to do this is with bio-identical thyroid, which is a combination of T3 and T4 (our bodies produce mostly T4 in the thyroid gland, send it out to the body where it is converted into T3, the active form). Bio-identical thyroid hormone is created to mimic the human hormone exactly, so the body can use it most efficiently. Many compounding pharmacies offer bio-identical thyroid.

Natural support for thyroid includes iodine, which is needed for the production of thyroid hormones (T3 has three molecules of iodine; T4 has four). Iodine is contraindicated in Hashimoto's thyroiditis, however, as it may trigger an autoimmune attack. Herbs such as bladderwrack and kelp boost thyroid, as does the amino acid tyrosine. The nutrients zinc and selenium are necessary for the healthy conversion of T4 to T3 in the body.

Reproductive hormones are also impacted by hypothalamic-pituitary dysregulation. Many men experience a drop in testosterone levels with chronic illness, and this contributes to loss of libido, sexual dysfunction, muscle weakness, loss of stamina, depression and sleep interruption. While herbs such as tribulus, maca and yohimbe can be potent tonics for men and help the situation, quite frequently a bio-identical testosterone supplement is best to normalize levels and improve function.

Any time reproductive hormones are out of balance or low, it is important to look at the adrenals. In both men and women, the adrenal glands are responsible for producing approximately 35-50% of the reproductive hormones estrogen, progesterone and testosterone. It follows that exhausted adrenals are not producing adequate levels of those as well as cortisol. Supporting adrenal function can improve symptoms that are related to reproductive hormones, too.

Lyme typically follows a pattern of four-week flares, even in men. However, in women, the flares usually coincide with the menstrual cycle, creating a double whammy. PMS symptoms can be severe in combination with the flare of general Lyme symptoms. And chocolate is off the list as a coping mechanism!

Herbs to support progesterone function such as Vitex (chaste tree) can be helpful. Some women do well with bio-identical progesterone in the second half of their menstrual cycle to lessen the severity of PMS.

For menopausal women, black cohosh, red clover, licorice root and other more estrogenic herbs are indicated along with the chaste tree. Anecdotally, I have found black cohosh to be helpful for the bladder irritation associated with Lyme disease in any gender and age group.

The night sweats of Babesia can be confusing for a woman of menopausal age, as often doctors attribute that symptom to their hormones when it may in fact be infection related. Sometimes both factors play a role, and both need to be addressed. Bio-identical hormone support with estrogen, progesterone and/ or testosterone can be hugely beneficial to women with chronic Lyme disease.

Pain Management

Pain management is a huge issue in Lyme disease as pain is present in some form for most people. There are different types of pain and causes of pain. Sometimes pharmaceutical pain management is necessary while a person is undergoing treatment to make pain levels manageable. Natural approaches may be enough for some while others may need complement medications.

Joint and Muscle Pain

Magnesium is one of the best natural remedies for muscle pain. Magnesium relaxes skeletal muscle so it can help take away some of the tightness of painful, aching muscles. Epsom salts baths contain magnesium sulfate, and this is why they too can cause easing of muscle pain (some people who are sensitive to sulfates or sulfur compounds may feel worse with Epsom salts baths). Magnesium's relaxing effect also works on smooth muscle. Since the intestinal wall contains smooth muscle, magnesium is an effective treatment for constipation.

Malic acid is good for muscle pain too, working through a slightly different mechanism. Research has shown that muscle pain with chronic illnesses such as Lyme and fibromyalgia is associated with low muscle tissue oxygen pressure in the affected muscles. This hypoxia results in a low output of ATP in the muscle cells. Essentially, this represents a block in the energy production cycle, which malic acid can overcome.

Some of the herbal anti-inflammatories, which include white willow and holy basil, work well for joint pain and muscle pain. Curcumin, which is found in turmeric, has well-researched anti-inflammatory activity.

Proteolytic enzymes can modulate inflammation by helping to break down some of the chemical mediators and tissue by-products. These are not digestive enzymes, which are taken with food to assist in digestion, but are systemic enzymes that are deliberately taken away from food to allow their uptake into the blood stream and through the tissues. Examples of these are bromelain, papain and protease.

Another pain modulating remedy, which requires a prescription from a compounding pharmacy, is Low Dose Naltrexone (LDN). LDN is an immune modulator, meaning it balances immune function. For this reason, it is used not only in conditions of low immunity but also in autoimmune issues such as rheumatoid arthritis and Hashimoto's thyroiditis. It has a mild blocking effect on opioid receptors in the brain, which stimulate the body to upregulate its production of both enkephalins (immune balancing chemicals) and endorphins (feel good chemicals). It has one negative side effect of a transient sleep disturbance, which occurs in one or two people out of ten (based on my clinical observations), but there is a subset of people for whom LDN gives great pain relief and enhances overall feelings of well-being.

Nerve Pain

Lyme patients often suffer from nerve pain, which can be burning, shooting or stabbing, and can range from mild to debilitating.

Some people get relief from nerve pain with methyl-B12 injections. B12 has a long track record of being used to treat neuropathy; some find it helps with the neuropathic pain also.

Herbs that can offset nerve pain include St John's Wort, Jamaica dogwood, lemon balm and skullcap. Curcumin can be helpful here too, both internally and in topical preparations.

Sleep

Sleep disturbance is one of the more common symptoms in Lyme disease. It is a catch-22 situation, since sufficient duration and quality of sleep is critical for the body to heal, and yet good quality sleep is often elusive for Lyme sufferers.

Natural aids for sleep can be helpful. Melatonin is a hormone that we produce naturally to regulate our day/ night, light/ dark cycles. Melatonin can safely be supplemented and can aid in falling asleep; however it has a short span of activity and is less effective for sleeping through the night. Sustained release melatonin is available and would be a better choice for that.

5-HTP is an amino acid precursor to serotonin, and in higher doses can assist sleep. Up to 200mg at night is needed. Herbs for sleep include valerian, passionflower, chamomile, skullcap and California poppy. We have found that combinations of the above work better and have formulated Dr. Nicola's Sleep Support in response to that.

Epsom salts baths at night have proved helpful for relaxing both the muscles and the mind.

Mood

Lyme disease impacts moods, which can present as anything from mild depression, irritability or anxiety to paranoid thinking and obsessive-compulsive traits. Mood changes in Lyme can be looked at from two viewpoints. The first is that Lyme disease is a painful, life-changing, often debilitating illness; with very little information or acknowledgement from the medical community; limited understanding even from the most well-meaning family and friends; and until recently very little support or hope. It is quite natural, in the light of all that, to feel depressed, anxious and even quite hopeless.

The second is that Borrelia and co-infections do infect the brain and do have a physiological impact on both neurotransmitters and brain wave patterns. Neurotransmitters are the chemicals created in our central nervous systems that regulate our thoughts, moods, behaviors and cognition. These infections directly impact the brain and subsequently impact moods as well.

So the problem is twofold—the infections themselves create mood and personality changes. Then there is the very valid issue of the mental and emotional struggle to cope with a crippling and highly misunderstood illness.

Modulating neurotransmitters can be helpful to balance moods, and can be done through use of specific amino acids that provide the building blocks for the neurotransmitters.

5-HTP is one of the key supplements used because it supports serotonin, which is a calming brain chemical (we call it an inhibitory neurotransmitter). This is the first choice in depression. GABA and theanine are indicated for states of anxiety. If obsessive-compulsive traits are presenting (as they often do in Bartonella cases), inositol in high doses (5-10 grams) may take the edge off. Where depression is more an exhaustive state, with no physical or mental energy, tyrosine can be helpful as it fuels dopamine, epinephrine and norepinephrine, which are more energizing and stimulating neurotransmitters. Tyrosine has an added benefit of supporting thyroid function (low thyroid function is a cause of depression, too).

Heavy Metal Toxicity

One thing I see more and more is Lyme disease patients with high levels of toxic metals such as lead and mercury.

Toxic metals can come from a variety of sources. Lead, while more strictly regulated today, used to be found in pencils, petrol, paint and pipes, to name a few. Older houses can still be sources of lead. Mercury can be found in vaccines, amalgam fillings and seafood. Both metals are inherent in pollution—both air and water—and so we all take in a certain amount of toxic metals daily. Coal burning power plants are a major source of mercury and other air-borne toxins. Aluminum, cadmium and arsenic are other metals that can accumulate in the body and cause problems. In fact, research shows a link between aluminum levels in the brain and Alzheimer's disease.

High levels of toxic metals in the system can cause neurological problems such as numbness, tingling and palsy as well as muscle aches, joint pain and cognitive dysfunction including memory loss and difficulty concentrating. It is easy to see how closely these symptoms resemble typical Lyme disease symptoms, and so an evaluation of whether toxic metals might be contributing to the Lyme disease picture is useful.

Not every Lyme patient has toxic metals, and not every person with toxic metals has Lyme disease. However, there does seem to be a correlation between Lyme disease and heavy metal toxicity. Recent research has also revealed that heavy metal toxins are often concentrated in the same parts of the body where Borrelia and co-infections make their home.

The question stands as to why Lyme disease patients are more impacted by heavy metals than other people in the population. My opinion is that Lyme patients have compromised detoxification mechanisms, and they are not able to rid themselves of heavy metals as they come into the body; hence, an accumulation occurs.

Lyme patients are also more neurologically stressed because they already have chronic infection impacting that system. So when another neurological stressor such as a toxic metal enters the picture, the impact is doubled.

Testing for Heavy Metals

There are a number of ways to test for heavy metals, each with its own merits and limitations.

Blood Test

This is the easiest and most readily available test through commercial laboratories. The problem with blood testing is that when metals come into the body, they only circulate in the blood stream for a period of a few weeks. After that they are taken up into the tissues—whether that be into the brain and neurological system, the joints and muscles, or the cardiovascular system (lead is implicated in cardiovascular disease through its presence in blood vessels and contribution to atherosclerosis). Therefore, unless there is a recent exposure to toxic metals, blood tests may well come back normal, completely missing the impact of metals already in the tissues.

Unprovoked Urine Test

An unprovoked urine test is a urine collection done without any pro-voking agent given beforehand. Again, this is a simple test to do, but the problem is that the urine is simply a filtration of the blood. There-fore an unprovoked urine test is going to carry the same limitations as blood testing. As with the blood, this test can be helpful if there has been a known recent exposure to metals, such as amalgam fillings being removed without proper precautions being taken to protect the body from mercury vapor. In cases of long-standing metal toxicity, it will be of limited benefit.

Provoked Urine Test

In many cases this is my preferred test. In this case, the patient is "provoked" with a dose of a heavy metal chelator prior to collect-ing the urine. Typically DMSA, an agent that bonds to the metal and "escorts" it out of the body, is used. DMSA is an agent that is known to chelate (bind) mercury in particular, and to a lesser extent, lead and other toxic metals.

The provoking agent serves to push the metals out of the tissues and back into the blood stream where they can be filtered by the kidneys. With a six-hour urine collection, levels of many different metals can be measured.

Granted, while this test is measuring how much toxic metal is dumped after a single dose of DMSA, it does not measure remaining body stores. However, we know that high levels of metals in the body correlate with high levels being dumped in the urine, because as we repeat the same test using the same provocation every two months, and as metals are chelated out of the body, we see the amount dumped with the provocation lessening over time. This indicates that the heavy metal detox protocol is working.

In some cases we do an unprovoked urine test first, then do a provoked one after the dose of DMSA and compare the results to determine how much of the heavy metal burden is from recent exposure versus body tissue stores. For the provoked test, all urine excreted over a six-hour period is collected, with a small sample of that sent back to the lab.

Caution must be taken with patients who are very chronically and severely ill because the provocation dose may cause a detoxification reaction that could set them back. Heavy metals when mobilized can cause headaches, joint and muscle pain, fatigue and neurological problems—the body's detoxification mechanisms must be functioning adequately to handle this. Furthermore, there is the possibility that the chelator used for provocation, such as DMSA, may actually cause metals to be redistributed throughout the body, sometimes to more sensitive locations (such as the brain and liver) than their original storage sites.

The majority of people can tolerate the provoked metals test. In more sensitive patients we can reduce the dose of DMSA, slightly reducing the benefit of the test but also protecting them from severe detox reactions. There is a subset of patients who are too sick and too sensitive to safely carry out this test. In such cases, I will either do an unprovoked urine test or a hair analysis.

Hair Analysis

I am not a strong advocate of hair testing for heavy metals, but this can be a valid starting point in patients who are too sensitive to do the provoked urine test. It is an easy and non-invasive test since it only requires a hair sample; however, there can be inherent challenges in the interpretation of the results.

If a person's hair showed a high level of metals, it could indicate that they are metal toxic and have a lot to excrete. However, if a person is showing low levels of metals in the hair, one could argue that they are unable to adequately excrete them and still have them in their system. Also, the hair test may be skewed by contaminants such as hair dyes and styling products.

I use the hair analysis in patients where we do not feel they could tolerate the urine test or in very small children, and in some cases it provides useful information. However, it is not my first choice for heavy metal assessment.

Addressing Heavy Metals

There are a number of ways to address heavy levels, and treatment choices should be made based on the severity of the problem, as well as how ill the patient is and how sensitive they are. A Lyme disease patient who has debilitating symptoms and shows extreme Herx reactions with any new modality should be treated very gently, while a more functional person with some symptoms but a generally good tolerance can be treated more aggressively. It should be noted that detoxifying heavy metals can be a high-risk proposition, as these metals are extremely damaging to all systems of the body and they can end up being redistributed throughout the body if chelation protocols are not carried out correctly.

A viable starting point for heavy metal detox is to dose with an agent that binds metals without actually stirring up tissue stores too much. Chlorella, a single-cell green algae, is probably the best-known example of this and is sometimes used to bind up biotoxins in Lyme disease also.

Cilantro is a herb that has been used for heavy metal detox. It has the ability to mobilize tissue stores of toxic metals so it may cause more of a detox reaction than chlorella alone. Cilantro is known for its ability to mobilize metals from the brain.

DMSA has been mentioned as we often use it as the provoking agent for urine metals tests. It preferentially pulls mercury but will also chelate lead and other metals such as aluminum and cadmium.

EDTA is another well-known chelating agent that has a stronger affinity for lead. It is not typically given orally as is DMSA, but instead either intravenously or via rectal suppository.

Other natural agents used to heavy metal detox include alpha-lipoic acid, high dose vitamin C, garlic and zeolite.

My preferred regimen for heavy metal detox in Lyme disease patients is a slow and steady approach, one that will not overwhelm the system, add stress to the detoxification processes or cause any worsening of symptoms. I use a product called Chelex (made by Xymogen) that has small amounts of DMSA and EDTA, combined with cilantro, chlorella, garlic and alpha-lipoic acid. It can be taken every day without risk of depleting minerals, or every second or third day for an even more gentle approach.

For those who want or need a more rigorous protocol, DMSA or EDTA is used depending on which toxic metal showed to be more problematic on the provoked urine test. Cyclic dosing schedules are created, balancing stronger chelating protocols with mineral repletion.

One thing that is true of any heavy metal detox program is that fibers and binders are crucial to make sure the metals that are being dumped into the bowels via the bile are being excreted, and not reabsorbed into the blood stream and redistributed to the brain. Chlorella is helpful here, but adding fibers such as psyllium husk, ground flax seed, bentonite clay or apple pectin may be necessary.

Heavy metal toxicity is something that all Lyme patients should evaluate at some stage of their recovery. For many, it is not the primary priority—getting adequate Lyme treatment should be the first priority, and often with the amount of medications and supplements required for that, and the energy required to handle the Herxing, there is not a lot left over to deal with anything else! Patients on more established regimens that have had some improvement and are managing their Lyme disease protocol well might be better positioned to examine the toxic metal issue. Heavy metal detox should be done under the supervision of a health practitioner with expertise in this area, as doing it the wrong way or too quickly can make things worse.

■ ■ ■ ■

As you can see, there are many natural ways to help support the immune system, manage pain and inflammation, support digestion, balance hormones and eradicate pathogens using naturopathic therapies. The ones presented are just the ones I have primarily used and seen in my practice. There are literally hundreds of other tools and techniques in the world of natural medicine, and a wide variety of practitioners with unique expertise.

Sample Naturopathic Protocols

This list represents a sample of some of my favorite products that I use extensively in my practice. It does not necessarily cover all the individual ingredients listed, however it provides consolidated protocols that can be easily followed. Protocols using other products listed and respective dosages should be formulated on an individual basis in conjunction with a qualified naturopath. This list is not representative of a complete protocol, where every supplement is recommended. Specific supplements are selected depending on individual need.

I have worked with a master herbalist in the design of the RestorMedicine herbal formulas, and all come from either organic or wildcrafted herbs. Researched Nutritionals is a nutraceutical company based in California that designs formulas tailored to Lyme disease and other chronic illnesses, and I use their products because of their impeccable standards, the way they combine various nutrients so that protocols can be streamlined, and the efficacy of their products.

I have marked RestorMedicine products with * and Researched Nutritionals products with **. Full descriptions of products and ordering information is available at www.restormedicine.com. This information is reprinted in Appendix H.

Detoxification Support

- Smilax *   40 drops twice daily
- Detox Support Formula *   40 drops twice daily
- Tri-Fortify Glutathione **   1 teaspoon in the morning in water
- Dr. Nicola's Detox Plus Powder *   2 scoops daily

Immune Support

- Transfer Factor Multi-Immune **   2 capsules before bed
- Transfer Factor LymPlus **   2 capsules before bed

Digestive Support

- RestorProbiotic Powder *   ½ - 1 scoop before bed
- (or) Prescript Assist **   2 capsules at night before bed
- Dr. Nicola's Fiber Plus *   4 capsules at night
- Anti-Parasite Formula *   40 drops three times daily
- Anti-Fungal Formula *   40 drops three times daily

Pain and Inflammation

- Soothe and Relaxx **   3 capsules twice daily
- InflaQuell **   3 capsules twice daily between meals
- Nerve Pain Formula *   40 drops three or four times daily

Mood and Sleep

- Soothe and Relaxx **   3 capsules twice daily
- Dr. Nicola's Sleep Support *   2 to 4 capsules before bed
- 200mg of Zen (ARG)   2 capsules twice daily
- 5-HTP   50mg   1 twice daily for mood; up to 4 before bed for sleep

Cognitive Function

- Tri-Fortify Glutathione ** 1 teaspoon in the morning in water

- Cognicare ** 2 twice daily

Adrenal Support (Energy)

- Energy Multiplex ** 3 capsules in the morning
- Licorice Plus (Metagenics) 2 tablets twice daily
- Adreset (Metagenics) 1 capsule twice daily
- DHEA Plus (Douglas Labs) 1 capsule daily in the morning

Mitochondrial Support (Energy)

- ATP Fuel ** 5 capsules twice daily
- CoQ10 400mg ** 1 capsule daily
- Ribos-Cardio ** 1 scoop daily

Antimicrobial

- Teasel Root * 5 drops twice daily
- Lyme Support Formula * 10 drops twice daily
- Artemisinin SOD ** 2 capsules twice daily
- HH2 Formula (Zhang) 1 capsule three times daily

Biofilm

- Boulouke Lumbrokinase ** 1 capsule twice daily between meals

- InflaQuell ** 3 capsules twice daily between meals

- Interfase Plus (Klaire Labs) 2 capsules twice daily between meals

Heavy Metal Chelation

- Chelex (Xymogen) 4 capsules one or two times daily
- DMSA 250mg (Thorne) 1 capsule three times daily, 3 days on/ 7 days off
- EDTA 750mg (compounded) 1 suppository every other night
- Multiple Mineral (Klaire Labs) 2 capsules on non-DMSA/ non-EDTA days

REFERENCES

1. Ionescu G, Kiehl R, Wichmann Kunz F, et al. Oral citrus seed extract in atopic eczema: in vitro and in vivo studies on intestinal microflor. J Orthomol Med. 1990;5(3):155-57.

16. NUTRITION AND LYME DISEASE

LYME DISEASE SUFFERERS WHO PAY ATTENTION TO THEIR NUTRITION and make positive dietary changes invariably do better than those who do not. The right diet can make such a huge contribution to recovery and level of symptoms. If nothing else, dietary modification is necessary while on antibiotic protocols to help prevent the yeast issues that can arise along the way, but food can truly be used as medicine.

I feel so passionately about this topic, and my patients were so eager for information on it, that I wrote a book about it. For detailed information on The Lyme Diet, including practical applications, meal suggestions, acid/alkaline food lists and gluten-free food lists, I would refer you to my book, *The Lyme Diet: Nutritional Strategies for Healing from Lyme Disease.*[1]

What you will find below is an overview of the principles of The Lyme Diet including enough information to get you started and help you along the right nutritional path. My goal here is for you to see clearly how diet plays into your Lyme disease, and the ways in which changing your diet can help Lyme disease.

Inflammation

One of the key things nutrition can do is help moderate inflammation in the body. Lyme disease creates a lot of inflammation, which can fuel pain and swelling. Inflammation involves a complex cascade of processes, but the immune system and the chemicals it produces modulate much of it.

Inflammation can be systemic, all over the body, or localized to a specific area, as would be the case with an injury to a certain body part. In Lyme patients, inflammation can relate to joints, muscle tissues, the brain, cranial nerves or the tissues surrounding the heart, to name just a few.

Fats can be inflammatory or anti-inflammatory through their conversion to certain chemicals called prostaglandins. There are different types of prostaglandins (PGs): PG1 inhibits inflammation and has beneficial effects; PG2 has the direct opposite effects and fuels inflammation; while PG3 is a mixture of the two (but is thought of as more anti-inflammatory).

To reduce inflammation in the body we must promote PG1 formation and inhibit PG2 formation. Therefore we must choose foods that boost PG1 and avoid foods that boost PG2.

Saturated fats and trans fatty acids definitely fuel inflammation by increasing PG2 production and should be avoided.

Saturated fats are found in nature but are labeled the "bad fats." These include red meat and dairy products. Trans fatty acids are processed chemically altered fats such as margarine and shortening. They are found in "junk food" such as chips, pastries and candies.

This means that eating a lot of red meat, and any processed foods and deep fried foods, is going to worsen inflammation.

To reduce inflammation we want to choose fats that fuel PG1 production. These are the unsaturated fats, also called essential fats, containing omega-3 fatty acids. These are found in nature and have great health benefits. They are the "healthy fats."

Omega-3 fatty acids are perhaps the most important to deliberately take in the diet. They have the strongest anti-inflammatory effects, as well as being very important for neurological function. Omega-6s and omega-9s are important too, but come more easily through the regular daily diet.

Omega-3 fatty acids are contained in flax oil and fish oil. I recommend two to four grams of either one of these (or a mixture) every day. A good way to get this is to put one tablespoon of flax oil in a smoothie or on a salad; then take a supplement of two grams of fish oil. Fish oil has the added benefit of being high in DHA, another important and healthy fat.

The other key to reducing inflammation is to reduce inflammatory foods. Gluten and dairy are both inflammatory in nature. It is thought that many people are gluten intolerant and are unaware of it, as they do not always show pronounced digestive symptoms.

Gluten is found in wheat, oats, rye and barley, and is a hidden ingredient in many foods. Many people have trouble digesting the proteins in gluten, and it often triggers an immune reaction, leading to more inflammation. Gluten intolerance can also be an autoimmune process and can actually trigger the body's immune system to attack its own tissues including the brain. With all the immune problems inherent in Lyme disease, it makes sense that we want to lessen what the immune system has to deal with. Taking gluten out of the diet can relieve the immune system and the digestive system and create a much better picture of health.

Since gluten is contained in grains, it is typically found in carbohydrate foods such as breads and pastas. Lyme disease sufferers do best by avoiding too many carbohydrates anyway because of their inflammatory properties and the potential yeast overgrowth, so there is a dual benefit to avoiding them, and consequently gluten.

Many of my patients noticed a pronounced difference in how they feel when they removed gluten from their diets, and I highly recommend it.

Another food group that can cause inflammation is dairy. Dairy proteins found in milk, cheese, yoghurt, cottage cheese, etc. are not easy for humans to digest. They can trigger immune reactions, and create mucous in the body. Anyone with respiratory conditions such as chronic sinus issues or asthma should definitely avoid dairy—but there is good reason for Lyme patients to avoid it too, or at least minimize it. Since yoghurt is fermented, it is somewhat easier to digest than milk or cheese; and goat dairy is easier to digest than cow dairy (sheep dairy is somewhere in the middle but closer to cow dairy).

Finally, any food that a person is sensitive to can fuel inflammation. In a full-blown food allergy, the reaction to the offending food is usually immediate and obvious. Most people know what their allergens are and avoid those foods. However, there are different types of food reactions, called food sensitivities or intolerances. They are mediated by different immune cells that can cause more subtle or hidden reactions, sometimes taking up to 72 hours from ingesting the food to manifest. The food sensitivities are caused by IgG immune cell reactions, while food allergies are triggered by IgE immune reactions.

To evaluate food sensitivities it is possible to do an elimination and challenge test. To do this, all the most common allergens are removed from the diet for a period of 21 days (gluten, dairy, soy, eggs, corn, citrus, peanuts). During that period of time the immune system has the chance to rest, recover and reset (when the foods are being eaten every day, typically the immune system cannot even register a problem as it is being constantly bombarded). After 21 days, foods are reintroduced one by one and any reactions noted. Usually after the 21 days of rest, the reactions to any problematic foods will be much stronger and more obvious, and therefore easier to identify.

The elimination diet requires a fair bit of discipline and effort, and it still has the potential to miss foods that might not have been excluded for the 21 days but are still causing problems. I have had patients with IgG sensitivities to garlic, bananas and pineapple—not things that we would typically consider problematic. Therefore the best way to assess for IgG food sensitivities is through a blood test. This testing is available through labs such as Great Plains Laboratory and US Biotek, but as a word of warning, many medical doctors and allergists do not regard it as valid, so ask either an integrative or more open-minded medical doctor to order the tests for you!

Immunity

Many discussions have focused on immune function. Remember, your ability to fight Lyme depends on (1) your immune function, and (2) your ability to detoxify.

Nutrition can give immune function a boost. Fresh vegetables should be a large part of the diet. Vegetables contain vitamins, minerals and antioxidants, all of which the body needs in plentiful amounts. These nutrients facilitate cell growth and repair, cell-to-cell communication and metabolic processes. Enzymes in the body function to catalyze, or speed up, all of our biochemical reactions. Nutrients such as B vitamins, zinc and magnesium are required for those pathways to operate efficiently.

Green leafy veggies may well be the healthiest, but I suggest a broad range of colors. Different colored vegetables contain different proportions of vitamins and minerals. A variety will ensure the best possible range.

High quality proteins are also important for immune function. Amino acids, the final breakdown product of proteins, are the building blocks of the body. Every cell and every tissue uses amino acids, including the immune system. High quality proteins include fish, chicken, some red meat (grass-fed red meat is ideal as it has a healthier fat content), eggs, nuts and seeds. This is one of the reasons I suggest a protein smoothie in the morning, to provide good quality proteins for the immune system to use. High quality proteins also keep the blood sugar stable and support adrenal function, which will in turn help the immune system.

The other part of supporting immunity is to avoid foods that suppress it. The main culprit in immune suppression is sugar. Studies have shown that one teaspoon of sugar can suppress immune function for up to 16 hours.

The mechanism by which sugar suppresses immune function involves insulin, the hormone that functions to shuttle sugar out of the blood and into the cells. When we eat sugar, insulin is released. The more sugar we eat, the more insulin is released. Insulin can circulate in the bloodstream long after the sugar has been metabolized, and an unwanted side effect of that is that the release of growth hormone from the pituitary gland is suppressed. Growth hormone is necessary for repair and recovery to occur in the body, and it is also a regulator of immune function. Therefore when sugar is eaten constantly, there is a constant flood of insulin in the blood stream, which in turn affects pituitary output of growth hormones and can create an immune deficiency.

Between the immune dampening and yeast-promoting effects of sugar, it is clear that Lyme patients are better off avoiding it altogether.

Digestion

There are several ways that nutrition can help digestive function. We already discussed that it is important to have gut function working optimally when treating Lyme disease—it is crucial to have a bowel movement at least once every day. If the bowels are sluggish and constipation is an issue, a high fiber diet along with supplementation with magnesium and vitamin C if necessary should be adopted to override this.

Fiber can also be used to sweep the bowels and clear toxins out. This is essential during antimicrobial therapy for Lyme and also during heavy metal detoxification.

As already discussed, good fibers for this are ground flax seeds and psyllium husk. I suggest a tablespoon of ground flax seeds in a protein smoothie every morning. Some people add flax seeds to salads or yoghurt. They must be ground, however, as whole flax seeds will pass through the intestinal tract without having the same sweeping effect as the ground ones. Psyllium husk is a little "rougher" than flax and does not contain the same cancer-preventing lignans, however for constipation it might be more effective.

Vegetables provide a great source of insoluble fiber. This is yet another reason to eat lots of fresh vegetables. Fruits contain more soluble fiber and they are beneficial too, but most Lyme patients restrict fruits because of their sugar content.

Candida, the naturally occurring yeast in the gut that tends to get overgrown during antibiotic therapy, feeds on sugar. All yeasts feed on sugar. One of the most fundamental principles of The Lyme Diet is to reduce sugar and carbohydrates, so as not to give the yeast a fuel source.

Avoiding sugars means not eating any refined sugars such as chocolate, candies, cakes, ice cream, etc. But it also means being mindful of all carbohydrates, even the "healthy" ones, as ultimately all carbohydrates break down into sugars. This includes fruit and whole grains.

Most of us have been brought up with the belief that fruit is a "good for you" thing, and in many ways it is. It is packed with vitamins and minerals and soluble fiber, and it is all-natural. However, fruit is also a source of sugar, mainly fructose, and this too can feed yeast. For my patients with existing yeast issues, typically it is necessary to remove fruit from the diet for a period of time; for those without yeast issues but who still need to be mindful of prevention, one to two pieces a day is the limit.

Bear in mind that Candida and Lyme disease tend to go hand in hand, regardless of whether one is on antibiotics or not. In other words, many people with Lyme still struggle with Candida issues even when not taking antibiotics. Subsequently these guidelines apply to all Lyme patients.

The other way to foster good digestion is to avoid those food allergens and intolerances that we discussed in the section on inflammation. Any food that causes an immune reaction in the gut will cause some problems, whether or not they manifest overtly as digestive symptoms. Gas, bloating, constipation and diarrhea are all possible symptoms of food intolerances.

Foods that cause inflammation in the gut can also lead to leaky gut. This is where the cells in the small intestine spread out, allowing larger than normal food particles to enter the blood stream. We discussed this in the section on naturopathic treatments for Lyme disease and gave some suggestions for gut-healing nutrients. Fundamental to improvement is removing the offending foods that are causing the problem in the first place—that is, gluten, dairy and any other foods that trigger an IgG food sensitivity reaction.

Detoxification

Have you gathered by now the importance of detoxification for a Lyme patient?! We can help our detoxification pathways by the foods that we eat and those we avoid.

The liver, the primary organ of detoxification, is responsible for trapping toxins, converting them to less harmful forms and preparing them for excretion from the body. One of the kindest things we can do for our liver is simply to minimize the intake of toxins to reduce the load with which it has to cope.

This means eating organic fruits and vegetables whenever possible. It also means eating free-range meats, poultry and eggs—where the birds and animals have been raised without hefty doses of hormones and antibiotics. Remember, if they were fed antibiotics and hormones, residues of those will be entering your body when you eat them.

I understand that eating all organic produce and free-range or grass-fed meats and poultry can be expensive, and potentially more difficult to find. However, the reward is that the liver has a lighter load to carry, which can help the way you feel.

Fish is a contentious issue. I believe wild-caught fish to have a healthier fatty acid composition, however there are concerns about heavy metal levels. Mercury is a known neurotoxin and is terrible for Lyme patients. Farm-raised fish are often fed a grain diet and given medications along the way, so they are not really an ideal choice either. The best solution in my opinion is still to eat wild-caught fish, but to choose the types of fish that are lower on the mercury scale (such as salmon) and limit seafood intake to twice weekly.

Foods that promote liver detoxification include artichokes, onions, garlic, beets, broccoli, spinach, cabbage, Brazil nuts, asparagus, avocado, papaya and cayenne. Any processed foods drag the liver down and should be avoided.

The other crucial element for detoxification is water. Since water makes up such a large proportion of our bodies, we must be constantly taking in fresh clean water for its cleansing and hydrating effects. Municipal water is high in chlorine and can potentially contain toxic elements such as heavy metals. Having adequately filtered water is important to avoid these pollutants. Most people should drink two liters (approximately half a gallon) per day.

Adding lemon juice to water helps to alkalinize the body (counterintuitive perhaps since lemon juice seems so acidic, but the overall effect in the body is alkaline), and to detoxify. The juice of one lemon squeezed into warm water is a good way to start the day, and is especially indicated during Herxes. Herbal teas are a good way to take in more water in a more holistic way while also naturally aiding various systems in your body. Peppermint helps digestive function, chamomile calms the nervous system, marshmallow soothes an inflamed gut, licorice helps adrenal function, dandelion root boosts liver detox and dandelion leaf is a natural diuretic and kidney tonic. That is only a small sample of the herbs with medicinal effects that can be taken as tea.

Summary of Nutritional Principles

For a Lyme sufferer, the emphasis should be on:

- Vegetables
- Lean proteins
- Healthy fats

While eating less:

- Fruits
- Carbohydrates
- Processed foods

As mentioned before, vegetables should contain a range of different colors. Baby spinach, capsicum (green, red and yellow), tomatoes, beans, cauliflower and broccoli are just a few examples.

Ideally, eat less of the root vegetables such as potatoes, carrots, turnips and beets as they are starchier and can have a greater impact on yeast.

Lean proteins include fish, chicken, turkey, lean red meat (no more than once or twice a week) and eggs. Again, I strongly advise meats from animals that have been raised without hormones and antibiotics. Meats from grass-fed animals (as opposed to grain fed) have been shown to have a much more beneficial fatty acid profile. That is, they have less saturated fat (which as you remember are the ones that fuel inflamma-tion). Historically, even beef contained healthy omega-3 fats, but when the cattle were taken off the fields, placed into stalls and fed a man-made, processed diet, their fat content became much more saturated, which was detrimental to the health of those who ate their meat.

Vegetarians will rely on tofu and legumes for their protein, and are strongly advised to drink a protein smoothie every day. In fact, everyone is strongly advised to drink a protein smoothie every day!

Healthy fats include the flax and fish oils discussed as anti-inflammatory oils, but there are also healthy fats found in avocado, olives and olive oil, and raw nuts and seeds.

Flax and olive oil are my preferred oils when used at room temperature or refrigerated, such as in salad dressings. For cooking, however, these oils will go rancid at higher temperatures, which counteract their health benefits. I recommend coconut oil for cooking, as it is stable at high temperatures. Coconut oil has two other benefits: It contains lauric acid, which is immune boosting and antiviral; and it contains caprylic acid, which is antifungal. While coconut oil was traditionally classified a satu-rated fat, it has a slightly different molecular structure to other saturated fats (containing medium chain triglycerides) which gives it more health benefits.

Foods to Avoid

As we have seen, fruits should not be eaten in abundance in Lyme dis-ease, mostly because of their sugar content and effect on Candida. One or two pieces a day are acceptable for a person with no known yeast issues; during antibiotic therapy I suggest a limit of one piece a day; and if known yeast problems exist, fruit may need to be completely excluded for a period of time.

Fruit does contain lots of good vitamins and minerals. However, a wide variety of vegetables will also provide that without promoting yeast.

For the same reason, carbohydrates such as pastas, breads, potatoes, and

rice may need to be restricted, as ultimately they get digested to s
and can impact yeast. The starchy carbohydrates I prefer include qu.....,
sweet potato and brown rice, mostly because they have a lesser impact
on blood sugar, but even these can feed yeast in a susceptible individual.
Decisions about how much fruit and starchy carbohydrates to eat are an
individual one based on Candida, blood sugar and energy levels. Generally speaking those on antibiotics need to be stricter than those who are
not, however I have seen both groups benefit from a low-carb diet.

Processed foods also need to be avoided. Full of saturated fats, hidden
sugars, high-fructose corn syrup and gluten, processed foods add little in
nutritional value to the diet. They can be a source of toxins and chemicals, and are rarely high in vitamins and minerals.

Drinks

The best fluids to take are water and herbal tea, approximately two liters
daily. Lemon juice in water is also a good drink.

My single favorite nutritional boost is the protein smoothie. I encourage
everyone to do a protein smoothie in the morning. The proteins provide
a steady source of energy and help keep blood sugar balanced, which in
turn helps the adrenal glands. A smoothie can also be a vessel for mixing
other nutrients such as flax oil, and even nutritional supplements.

My favorite recipe is:

1 cup almond or rice milk
1 scoop protein powder (such as brown rice protein,
whey protein, egg white protein, pea protein) *
1 tablespoon flax oil or coconut oil
1 tablespoon ground flax seed
1 cup fresh or frozen fruit (optional)

* Which protein powder to choose depends largely on your individual
sensitivities.

Whey, although a dairy product, can be acceptable for some people. In dairy, the two major proteins are casein and whey. Of the two, casein is the more problematic and harmful. Whey, once isolated and purified, can promote liver detoxification and provide a high quality protein. Food sensitivity tests should indicate whether one is sensitive to whey and eggs, and that will help guide choices. For our highly sensitive patients we use a blend of rice, pea and chlorella proteins, such as in our formulation Dr. Nicola's Detox Plus powder (which also contains nutrients to support detox and gut healing).

This is possibly the healthiest way to start your day providing not only proteins, but omega-3 fatty acids, fiber and lignans.

The other highly beneficial drink is a green smoothie. I am not a proponent of juices that are high in sugars such as fruits, and vegetables such as beets and carrots. I am also more of an advocate of high-powered blenders that completely liquefy vegetables, rather than juicers that extract the juice and leave all the beneficial fibers out. Not only is the fiber which benefits the bowels lost, the juice alone will transport through the gut and bloodstream more quickly without the effect of the fiber to slow it down, and can potentially have a detrimental effect on blood sugar. Vegetables such as spinach, cucumber and celery are good bases. Ginger and garlic can be added for flavor and their medicinal properties. I even add avocados to my green smoothies, and for those without major yeast issues who can do 1-2 pieces of fruit per day, a cup of berries or frozen mango sweetens it up.

Drinks to avoid are alcohol and coffee. Sorry about that.

Most Lyme patients become highly intolerant to alcohol, getting massive hangovers after only one drink. This typically provides enough of a deterrent. The liver, once again, is responsible for processing alcohol, so avoiding alcohol will remove one stressor, and that is worthwhile.

Lyme patients who are taking antibiotics should definitely avoid alcohol, as it can react adversely with the medications. Metronidazole (Flagyl), tinidazole and rifampin are particularly harsh so no alcohol should be consumed at all while on those medications.

The amount of alcohol in drop doses of herbal tinctures is minimal and should not trigger a reaction. However for more sensitive patients or those wanting to be really thorough, herbs can be put into hot water, which will evaporate off the alcohol, then cooled before drinking.

Coffee not only provides one more thing for the liver to process but also acts as a stimulant on the adrenals. It is tempting to use coffee for a quick energy boost given the fatigue that is so common in Lyme disease, but the boost is short lived, and ultimately it will add to exhaustion by taxing the adrenals. I am not categorically opposed to one cup of coffee a day, but if several cups are needed just to get through the day, that is a sign of a bigger adrenal issue that should be addressed.

Lifestyle Factors

Exercise

Whether or not to exercise is one of the common questions that arises for Lyme patients. For some, it is not even a possibility—walking to the bathroom and back seems too far and a momentous task. Fatigue, pain, dizziness, and neurological issues can be prohibitive, even to activities of daily living.

For others, especially for those who had a regular exercise plan prior to their illness, it may be beneficial to do some light exercise.

I believe that as long as the exercise does not exhaust you, and so long as it does not set you back for the next couple of days, it is acceptable. My rule of thumb is that if the activity feels good at the time and you feel good the following day, then it is okay.

I am also not opposed to aerobic activity, which raises the heart rate and pumps oxygen around the body. In some cases, this can be revitalizing, and healthy for the body. Again, the rules of thumb are to *listen to your body and if in doubt, go slow.*

Good forms of exercise for Lyme patients are walking, swimming, yoga, Pilates and light strength training (weights, dyna bands, Kettlebells etc.).

Running, tennis and other team sports are likely to be too intensive.

People with low cortisol need to be more careful as they have less fuel in the tank. Cortisol and the adrenals, among other things, are involved in the regulation of blood sugar. We think of insulin as the hormone responsible for this, and while that is especially true in the short term after we eat, cortisol also plays a significant role in the longer-term regulation of blood sugar. So people with erratic or insignificant cortisol production may be unable to adequately regulate their blood sugar post-exertion. The adrenals, through the hormone aldosterone, also play a role in salt and water balance in the body, and subsequently hydration. Poorly functioning adrenals may impact a person's ability to stay hydrated and maintain a healthy salt and water balance.

Those with low thyroid function, which is common in chronic Lyme disease, may struggle with exercise due to the fatigue and lethargy associated with it.

Hypoxia, or low oxygen in the muscle tissues, is often seen in both fibromyalgia and Lyme disease patients. This will make exercise all the more painful as there is not sufficient oxygenation in the muscle cells, the mitochondrial energy-production pathways are not able to create as much ATP (which requires oxygen), and muscles will feel fatigued and achy, even with the lightest exercise. My patients have told me that the day after taking a slow walk around the block, they felt like they had run a half marathon instead because of their muscle aches and pains. This is due to the lack of oxygen and ATP, coupled with a rapid accumulation of lactic acid that was not cleared out of the muscles due to their slow metabolic processes.

This is where magnesium and malic acid can be very helpful, as the malic acid helps to support the oxygenation of the muscles while the magnesium aids muscle relaxation.

Many people find that supplementing with ribose before a workout helps their strength and overall energy levels. Ribose is a five-carbon sugar, but it is not a "bad" sugar since it does not impact blood sugar negatively (in fact, some people find it actually gives them a lowering effect, and need to take it with food to offset this), and it does not feed Candida. It is a sugar that feeds skeletal muscle and cardiac muscle directly. Taken prior to exercise it can provide a fuel source for the muscles and promote endurance. Even without exercising, many people with chronic fatigue, muscle weakness and lack of stamina benefit from supplementing with ribose and malic acid.

Any of the mitochondrial support nutrients—NADH, CoQ10, L-carnitine, alpha keto-glutaric acid—can be helpful for supporting energy production and thus helpful for sustaining exercise.

As a disclaimer, supplements should not be used to "prop you up" in order to exercise. They can be aids but should not be crutches. If you require two shots of espresso to get out and walk around the block, but you could not walk that far yourself without the two shots, then you probably should not be doing it. Anything with a stimulant effect can be harmful, especially when taken over time. Stimulants, while they might feel good at the time, wear down your adrenals even faster and contribute to more profound exhaustion down the road.

For those who are very sick and bedridden, you may set a goal to do some arm lifts and leg lifts a couple of times a day, or to walk to the end of the driveway and back. Even if this is your limit, still try to do it a couple of times a day. If you are in a wheelchair perhaps you could use one or two-pound weights for some arm exercises.

Remember that the bugs do not like oxygen so increasing oxygen throughout the body is putting them at a disadvantage. Maintaining some mild gentle activity can be strengthening and rejuvenating for the body. It can also be a game-changer for mental outlook. Exercise has been shown to be among the most helpful interventions for depression, and understandably, many Lyme patients struggle with depression. Activity, at whatever level is comfortable for you, increases oxygen flow to the brain and boosts the happy chemicals such as endorphins, growth hormone and serotonin.

Sleep

Before I say anything about sleep, I want to acknowledge that many Lyme sufferers have tremendous sleep disturbance. I understand that my advice to get eight hours of sleep may frustrate you, because you would happily sleep for four hours if you could, but sleep is elusive. People with chronic Lyme disease tend to either sleep many hours at a time out of sheer and perpetual exhaustion, or the complete opposite occurs and they have trouble falling asleep, staying asleep, or both. Insomnia affects most Lyme sufferers at some stage of their illness.

In the section on naturopathic interventions we looked at some of the natural sleep aids that can be helpful. While I am not a fan of prescription sleep aids, there are times when they can be necessary in the short term to promote healthy sleep patterns.

The body does a lot of healing while we sleep. Cortisol levels fall at night (hopefully), and the immune system kicks up to do it's housekeeping. This is why symptoms sometimes feel worse at night, because the immune system is more active. This does not always hold true for all Lyme patients, partially because their immune system is operating on low levels to begin with, but it holds true for many.

The hours between 10pm and 2am are the most valuable hours in terms of physical regeneration. Therefore the more sleep you can get before midnight, the better off you are. Some people only need six hours sleep a night while others need eight or nine. Respect your body's need for sleep knowing it is using that time for healing. If in doubt, sleep more rather than less.

There are several things you can do to improve your sleep. Toxicity can be a major contributor to insomnia, so make sure your detoxification is sufficiently supported with smilax, glutathione, liver herbs, activated charcoal and so on. Magnesium sulfate (Epsom salts) baths at night are not only relaxing (the magnesium part) but they can give an extra boost to detox (the sulfate part).

Hormone imbalance also impacts sleep—low thyroid, while causing fatigue, can cause insomnia. Adrenal fatigue definitely impacts it, and many people find their sleep improves once their adrenals are better supported.

Electromagnetic fields can interfere with sleep patterns especially in highly sensitive people so remove as many electronic devices as possible from the bedroom, especially those with wireless or Bluetooth capabilities. Even getting rid of digital clock radios, cell phones by the bed, and cordless landlines makes a difference. A magnetic or earthing pad or sheet can offset the effects of electromagnetic fields.

Finally, create a cave for yourself. Get blackout curtains or blinds, have comfy bedding, make your bed a place you want to be. Have a protein snack before bed to keep your blood sugar stable through the night. And if sleep is elusive, make the decision that you will use that time to have productive, hopeful thoughts, not troublesome anxious ones. That might take some discipline at first, but the more you strengthen the neural pathways around positive thoughts, the easier it will be to draw on them.

REFERENCES

1. Ionescu G, Kiehl R, Wichmann Kunz F, et al. Oral citrus seed extract in atopic eczema: in vitro and in vivo studies on intestinal microflor. J Orthomol Med. 1990;5(3):155-57.McFadzean N. The Lyme diet: nutritional strategies for healing from Lyme disease. Legacy Line Publishing; 2010. 216 p.

17. CAN NATURAL THERAPIES ALONE TREAT LYME DISEASE?

I AM FREQUENTLY ASKED WHETHER IT IS POSSIBLE TO RECOVER from Lyme disease without the use of antibiotics. It's a great question, but unfortunately not one for which I have a definitive answer. Rather, my answer is "Sometimes." I wish I could tell people that they can treat their Lyme disease 100% naturally and have great outcomes every time, but that is just not realistic.

I definitely have patients that I work with without the use of antibiotics, where herbal antimicrobials and immune support, coupled with dietary changes and other supportive nutritional supplements have recovered them to the point where they are living their lives, either completely symptom free or at 90-95% of their normal (pre-Lyme) level of functioning. I love these cases as they really reinforce the power of natural medicine.

More often than not, when patients opt for all-natural treatment, it is necessary to select a variety of modalities to cover as many bases as possible. An example is to combine the immune-supportive properties of transfer factors (both general and Lyme-specific) with herbal antimicrobials (teasel, cats claw, olive leaf, etc) and Lyme-specific homeopathic remedies, and as I said, base all of that on a solid foundation of good nutrition. We want to address the infection from several directions at once to maximize the impact and our success. Of course supporting detoxification and digestive support are important, too.

197

In many cases herbs, nutrition and homeopathics will not be enough, and we need to step it up another notch. This is when I consider other therapies such as hyperbaric oxygen (HBOT). HBOT is a great way to improve oxygen flow to the cells, accelerating the cellular healing and regeneration. It also has antimicrobial action, as the bugs do not survive well in that high saturation of oxygen. It helps regenerate neurological function and sweeps the body of other microbes such as viruses and Mycoplasma. HBOT can be time and money intensive, and accessibility can be an issue, but it is a very valuable treatment option.

If HBOT is not an option, another approach is to engage some kind of Rife or frequency-based therapy. This is based on the premise that if the frequency of a certain pathogen is introduced to the body, that pathogen will be killed by the energy/ frequency that matches it. Rife machines can be purchased for home use, and some practitioners offer frequency-based therapy in their office. For more information on Rife therapy, see Bryan Rosner's book, *When Antibiotics Fail: Lyme Disease and Rife Machines*.

Alas, there are cases where antibiotics are necessary. I wish it wasn't so, but it is. Some people just can't recover sufficiently without these medications, and antibiotics offer relief that other more natural therapies cannot give. I honestly think that the majority of Lyme patients require antibiotic treatment at some time during their treatment. Of course, I always vote for naturopathic support in conjunction with the meds, and nutrition is equally if not even more important here. But the bottom line is that in many cases, medications are a necessary part of treatment.

There are a number of factors that determine whether a patient will respond well only to natural treatments. Duration of illness is one, as well as severity of symptoms. Obviously, a more recent case that hasn't gone as "deep" into the body will likely respond better. Also, I have had better success treating more naturally in cases where there is less neurological involvement. Arthritic-type Lyme seems to respond better to herbs and nutrient therapy, in part I believe because there are several great natural remedies for calming inflammation, which causes a lot of the pain. Minerals such as magnesium can offset a lot of the muscle aching, cramping and twitching.

So can Lyme disease be treated naturally? My answer is "Sometimes." My general philosophy is to start with natural agents and build up to medications if the patient is not responding adequately. At least then we have laid a solid foundation of support and started doing some bug-killing before the medications are introduced, and have set up detox pathways to function better and handle medications and die-off better. In medicine this is called the "therapeutic order"—start with the least invasive therapy and work up in strength and invasiveness as needed.

Another important part of this puzzle is to ensure other issues such as hormone imbalance, heavy metal toxicity, thyroid issues and food intolerances are being adequately addressed. Sometimes if Lyme symptoms are not resolving there is a tendency to get more and more aggressive with medications, adding new ones and increasing doses, when the problem may not be originating from the Lyme disease at all, and may be helped with something completely different such as gluten avoidance or chelation therapy.

Of course, Lyme disease is complicated. There is no answer that is right for everyone, and the thing that might be right for an individual today may not be right for them six months from now. A lot of the answers come from listening carefully to what the body is saying, and not being afraid to make adjustments as needed. Whether natural treatments or antibiotics are used, a multi-system, multi-factorial approach is the key to recovery from Lyme disease. We need to treat the person, not the disease.

SECTION FOUR

PUTTING IT
ALL TOGETHER

18. WHAT DOCTORS SHOULD KNOW ABOUT LYME DISEASE

IF YOU ARE A PHYSICIAN OR OTHER HEALTH PRACTITIONER READING this book, the first thing I want to say is "Thank You." Thank you for your openness, your willingness to learn, and your courage in stepping outside the status quo and recognizing that chronic Lyme disease is a real disease, and one that affects some, maybe many, of your patients.

There are a few key take-homes that I would like to emphasize for health-care providers.

1. The International Lyme and Associated Disease Society (ILADS) is a non-profit, multi-disciplinary, international medical society dedicated to disseminating accurate and practical information on Lyme and related illnesses. They hold annual conferences in the United States and in Europe, they have physician training programs and they publish treatment guidelines. Their website is www.ilads.org. They are a great resource for new doctors; in fact, they may be the most important resource in existence at the time of this book's writing.

2. Please consider Lyme disease when you have a patient with a multi-system illness, where traditional medical testing and imaging does not show a valid explanation for the symptoms. A trial of antibiotic therapy can provide useful diagnostic information (either through improvement or a flare of symptoms).

3. Patients often have no recollection of a tick bite or the typical EM rash. Lyme disease cannot be ruled out in the absence of these two things.

4. Lyme disease is a clinical diagnosis that can be made based on symptom picture and the patient's history. Lab work should be done to confirm the diagnosis and shed light on co-infections, but negative test results for Lyme do not rule out infection.

5. ELISA testing is not sufficiently sensitive to be considered reliable. Lab testing should be done through a specialist Lyme lab. IGeneX is the lab used by most Lyme-literate medical doctors in the United States and is considered the leader in the field of Lyme disease. Multiple test types should be run, including Western Blots, PCR and IFA for Borrelia; and antibodies and FISH tests for co-infections.

6. Lyme disease treatment protocols are complex and can be considerably different from standard antibiotic regimens. They are:

    - Long duration—several months up to two years and even beyond.
    - High dose—often these pathogens require higher than normal doses to be effective.
    - Multiple medications—medications must be combined to cover the three different life cycles of Borrelia—spirochete form, cell-wall deficient form and cyst form, as well as addressing co-infections along the way. The medications needed will vary throughout the recovery process, depending on which infection or infections are most active at any given point in time.

    These factors can make prescribing antibiotics for Lyme disease patients a challenging and intimidating task. Please continue to use this book, Dr. Burrascano's Advanced Topics in Lyme Disease and the ILADS Treatment Guidelines as resources (see Appendix A for Burrascano's 2008 Treatment Guidelines).

7. Recognize that the best approach to chronic Lyme disease is multidisciplinary. A team approach works well since no one practitioner can offer everything. A captain at the helm is always a good idea—one central doctor coordinating and overseeing the treatment—but recognizing when counselors, massage therapists, physical therapists, naturopaths and other allied health practitioners can be useful is a great bonus.

8. Please, please remain compassionate to the plight of Lyme disease patients. Please do not tell them they are crazy! Lyme patients need love and understanding and a kind, non-judgmental, listening ear. They have had way too many experiences of being cut off, dismissed, judged, ridiculed and shut down by other doctors. Please be the one that provides a different experience for them. None of us have all the answers, and Lyme disease is certainly a complex and challenging illness to treat. Sometimes, just being willing to listen and show compassion makes all the difference.

19. THE EMOTIONAL
CHALLENGES OF LYME DISEASE

LYME DISEASE NOT ONLY TAKES A HEFTY PHYSICAL TOLL ON THE body but exacts a great emotional toll as well. Here is just a sampling of some of the challenges inherent in the world of chronic Lyme disease:

Lack of diagnosis/ answers—"there's nothing wrong with you"

Most patients have seen many doctors in their quest for answers as to why they are so sick. This is mostly because doctors are not trained to recognize the symptoms of Lyme disease, nor run adequate tests for it. Often times many tests are run and studies undertaken, none of which return positive results, giving the appearance that there is nothing physically wrong with the person.

Further contributing to this problem is that in Western medicine today, the body has become so segregated. The nervous system is the domain of the neurologist, the bones are the domains of the rheumatologist, and the stomach is the domain of the gastroenterologist. The Primary Care Physician is the physician designed to know a bit about everything, but realistically their training has conditioned them to refer out to the specialists when their knowledge and experience bank is tapped. So many Lyme patients are sent to various specialists who are unable to diagnose the problems they are having in any given organ or system in isolation; they do not see the global picture. Even when the patient's symptoms do match the symptoms of disease patterns they are trained to look for, they might discharge the patient telling them that there is nothing physically wrong with them.

The diagnosis of psychosomatic symptoms—"it's all in your head" or worse "you're crazy"

It is very common for Lyme patients to be told that their illness is all in their head, that it is stress related or related to depression or anxiety. This is because in the slew of medical tests and studies performed in the evaluation of their illness, nothing really shows up to explain the symptoms. Coupled with this, Lyme patients are often depressed or anxious by the time they have been sick for years, seen multiple doctors, not gotten any real answers as to what might be happening to their bodies, and to top it off, have bacteria and parasites messing with their brain.

Most Lyme patients at some point in their illness have been offered or given anti-anxiety medications or anti-depressants from their doctor. I am not saying that there is not a place for these therapies in the treatment of chronic Lyme disease—sometimes they can be highly beneficial to stabilize the psycho-emotional aspects of the illness while treatment is undertaken. However, Lyme disease is a physical disease with psycho-emotional manifestations. It is *not* a psychiatric illness. Telling a Lyme patient they are crazy and need psychiatric help is cruel, misguided and unproductive. I am sure 100% of Lyme patients would opt for a healthy life and a healthy body if given the chance. They did not "choose" their illness or bring it on themselves. Granted, as is the case with any chronic illness, suffering can be a great teacher and many people learn a lot about themselves, which they would not have gained otherwise. I would also say that in some, there can be psycho-emotional barriers to healing, and when these elements are addressed, the body recovers faster. However, that is a very different position from the claim that Lyme patients are making up symptoms or that the illness is purely a manifestation of stress or anxiety.

Symptoms that are not always visible to the world—"but you look fine to me"

Many Lyme patients feel like death warmed over, but on the outside they look quite healthy. Joint pain, headaches, buzzing in the limbs, rapid heart rate, aching muscles, and shooting pains may not be visible to friends, colleagues and neighbors, even though to the person experiencing them, they seem to be taking over their entire being. Drenching sweats in the privacy of one's bedroom at night are not recognized by others in the light of day.

Lyme disease patients do not look like cancer patients who may have lost their hair or a lot of weight during chemotherapy. They do not appear as rheumatoid arthritis patients whose joints are so red and swollen that they are clearly visible to the outside world.

The agony of Lyme disease can be very isolating. Lyme patients often feel very misunderstood, and very alone in their illness. Lyme is especially hard on spouses and families. When Mom might not be well enough to take the kids to school or to play or help with homework, it puts strain on the household. It is not uncommon for spouses to question the validity of their mate's symptoms and illness, as often they do not present outwardly with the things we associate with illness such as weight loss, looking pale, deformities of the body, or other visible signs.

Lyme patients often have to "soldier on," maintaining jobs outside the home, keeping house and coordinating kids' schedules. At the same time, while they might appear to be holding it together, there is often incredible pain and suffering on the inside.

The unknown—"how long is this going to last?" and "will I ever really be well again?"

We do know that chronic Lyme disease requires long-term treatment. Rarely is it less than one year, often two years, and many times even longer than that. It makes it particularly hard to plan for, given the potential loss of income, and the expense of treatments, medications, supplements, doctor visits and so on. This long-term nature of treatment places tremendous strain on families—in ways that are both financial and non-financial.

The million-dollar question of "do we ever really cure Lyme disease?" is one that I am asked all the time. The current belief is that acute Lyme, if caught early (in the first few weeks) and treated aggressively enough, can be cured. Chronic Lyme, however, is believed to remain in the body on some level even with treatment. BUT—there is always the possibility of full recovery, and that is always the goal. Once levels of infection are lowered, the immune system should be able to handle the load on an ongoing basis. If you have had glandular fever, the virus that causes it (Epstein-Barr virus) is always going to be in your system. That does not necessarily mean that it will ever cause you problems again. Similarly, there are Lyme patients who have made a full recovery, and who may never again experience any Lyme symptoms. Granted, once the infection is treated, care still needs to be taken to maintain a healthy immune system through nutrition and lifestyle factors such as adequate sleep, stress management and so on; but recovery is possible and should always be the goal. Also, many patients are able to live a very normal life even if they have a few small remaining symptoms. Sometimes, recovery to 90% well, along with some ongoing maintenance treatments, is a large victory and will allow patients to resume their normal lifestyle and activities.

If Lyme patients maintain hope that they can and will recover, then they actually stand a greater chance of recovering (the profound power of the mind). One of the real barriers to this is trying to stay optimistic that recovery is possible in the light of information that the infection will never fully be cleared from the body. I believe that working on emotional blocks and negative thought patterns around this through therapies such as Emotional Freedom Technique (EFT) can help people overcome this emotional hurdle.

The multiple costs of the illness—"am I going to lose everything over this?"

The costs of Lyme disease are painfully high. I have known many to lose their homes, exhaust their savings, have to borrow from friends and family, and live on social security income because Lyme disease has ravaged their financial wellbeing. But the costs go way beyond finances. Many people have lost jobs that they loved; careers that they worked so hard for; hobbies and interests that gave them joy. Many marriages have crumbled as they simply could not withstand the stressors that come with such a misunderstood chronic illness. A few have even lost the ability to care for their children, and had to entrust them to friends, relatives or the state to provide what they could not.

The loss that can come with chronic Lyme disease is profound and can be devastating—years of lost income, friends lost through confusion and lack of understanding, loved ones lost through the challenges of trying to maintain a relationship. Many times there is a significant grief aspect to this illness that needs to be compassionately understood and addressed.

The guilt factor—"did I give this to my children?"

I believe that congenital Lyme exists. I have treated children of mothers who have Lyme disease, some of whom were exhibiting symptoms from a very young age; some of whom had a concurrent autism diagnosis; and some of whom have no record of a tick bite. The guilt a mother feels if there is any chance that she passed Lyme disease on to her child can be tremendous. Of course, many women did not know that they had Lyme disease when they were pregnant and breastfeeding, and how could they have? But now, they have sick children and they wish that they had had more information back then as well as an accurate diagnosis of their own, so that they could have made more informed decisions (such as taking antibiotics during pregnancy, not breastfeeding, etc). This provokes a lot of guilt, and also a lot of anger at the medical system for not providing answers when those answers could have made all the difference.

The experience of isolation—"am I all alone?"

One of the most difficult challenges for Lyme disease sufferers is the brick wall they face as soon as the words "Lyme disease" are mentioned. Doctors shut down, friends look blank, insurance companies close their checkbooks. Some deny that chronic Lyme exists and go on their merry way. Thankfully, some of the recent media coverage is extending knowledge of Lyme disease throughout the community, and people are recognizing themselves and their experiences in the stories they hear. Through the Internet, email groups are forming, information is being shared, and people are finding some solidarity in their newly formed "pack." Support groups are sprouting up in various areas, educational seminars are being planned, training programs are in development and more physicians are undertaking training with ILADS.

20. COPING STRATEGIES

Connie Strasheim, author of several books on Lyme disease including *Insights Into Lyme Disease Treatment: 13 Lyme-literate Practitioners Share Their Healing Strategies,*[1] also wrote a great book entitled *The Lyme Disease Survival Guide: Physical, Lifestyle and Emotional Strategies for Healing.*[2] I recommend this book to provide thoughts and ideas that will support you.

There are a collection of tools and habits that my patients have used that seem to make a difference and keep them moving forward. These are also things that I believe in as being able to make a contribution towards healing.

Create a network of support and positivity

From an emotional standpoint, a positive attitude and a strong support system is central to "surviving" the Lyme experience. Positive thoughts, positive actions and positive surroundings can make the difference between giving in to illness, and being able to face it head on each day, striving for a better future.

It is impossible to stay positive and hopeful when surrounded by negative and pessimistic people. Surrounding yourself with the right people who prop you up, encourage you, celebrate your victories, and empathize with your struggles without letting you get into a big pity party about them will boost your outlook and your healing. Create that environment deliberately. Sometimes it helps to be direct: Tell people what you need from them; tell them exactly what support looks like to you; tell them if you just want them to listen to you or if you want them to offer ideas or opinions; tell them what it provides for you when they give you encouragement and understanding. People often want to help but they do not know how. It is your job to let them know. They cannot read your mind.

Do not be afraid to let go of people who pull you down and who are constantly negative about you or your illness as they will hinder your recovery.

Where possible, and especially if you do not have a good support system at home or in your close surroundings, get a counselor or therapist whom you trust. They will always be there to support you and will provide you with compassion and understanding, which can be very healing. Just because a person has not experienced all you have experienced in your illness, does not mean they cannot be empathetic to what you are going through.

I have found Emotional Freedom Technique (EFT) to be a significant tool for patients. It is a technique that can be used to help release painful emotions. Once learned it can be done anywhere, anytime, and takes only a few minutes. It might be one of the best "coping tools" you can have in your arsenal. Another technique that is easy to do at home is binaural beat therapy (www.centerpointe.com). Listening to this CD daily helps the brain to reorganize itself into healthier patterns, leading to less anxiety and fear, better stress tolerance and a more positive outlook.

Also, do not be afraid to ask for help when the psychological and emotional aspects of the illness overwhelm you. Some people benefit from anti-depressant or anti-anxiety medications to get them through the hardest parts. You do not have to be a hero and suffer along needlessly. These medications, while I do not believe are the healthiest choice long term, can be life saving, or at least sanity saving, when used as a bridge to recovery.

Create an environment of positivity

Just as people can bring you up or down, so too can your environment make a big difference. Make sure to have things around you that represent freedom, health and wholeness. Do not pack your fishing gear or sporting equipment away in the back shed, assuming you will never be able to use them again. Keep them out. In fact, keep them handy (you may need them sooner than you think). The visual reminder keeps them in your present and future, not in your past.

I recommend people identify a few things that they enjoy doing and can manage, and do at least one every day. Examples are reading great books, talking to friends on the phone, listening to soulful music, sewing or writing—whatever are the things that you can do, do them. Even if it is just a few minutes each day, deliberately take time for something that brings you enjoyment.

Harness the Power of the Mind

Neuroscience is giving us amazing information about the brain that shatters all our preconceived notions. While once thought of as quite rigid and unchangeable, we now know that the brain is malleable. The term "neuroplasticity" has been coined to describe that phenomenon. What this means is that the brain is adaptable. If one part of the brain is damaged, a different part of the brain can take over its functions. That has been shown in conditions such as stroke, visual and auditory defects. It also means that the neural pathways can be shaped and strengthened, if we train them.

When we have a certain thought or thought pattern, which thought pattern travels along a neural pathway in the brain. There is both electrical activity and chemical activity associated with that. When we repeat that thought over and over again, the neural pathways representing it are strengthened. What started out as a "single lane dirt road" neural pathway can be grown and expanded into a "multi-lane superhighway" neural pathway. How? By repeated strengthening of that pathway, through repetition (the training effect). Given this information, it is easy to see that while positive thoughts may not seem like the easier ones to have in the midst of pain and illness, they are the ones you must have in order to strengthen those positive neural pathways. Giving in to chronic negative thinking will be a self-perpetuating, self-fulfilling prophecy—you will literally train your brain to think negatively, and that will manifest in your body.

This is incredibly powerful information that can be used to significantly influence your health. I would highly recommend two books on this subject—*Molecules of Emotion*[3] by Candace Pert and *The Brain That Changes Itself*[4] by Norman Doidge.

Dare to dream

It is ok to dream of the days when you will be well again. Imagine what they will be like, think about what you will do—where you will travel, who you will spend time with, what you will eat and drink, what you always wanted to do before but never had the time/ money/ motivation. There is nothing like a painful, debilitating illness to make you realize what is truly important to you and what really matters in life. Make wish lists, gather information on exotic destinations you would like to see, research saxophone lessons or read up on the breed of puppy that might work well for you. Whatever it is, dream it, with the plan of living it.

We know now that our reality follows our thoughts. What we think, we will create; it becomes our reality. We already see that we can choose our thoughts, but thoughts are also sourced from our imagination. I used the term "daydream on purpose" because that resonates for me—if we "daydream on purpose" we create those visions—we make them real in our minds—then our minds set to work on making them real in our lives. I used to think this was airy-fairy nonsense, but having studied the neuroscience behind it, I now see that this is very real, and that our dreams and imaginings are distinct predictors of our future.

Develop your spiritual connection

Everyone has different religious and spiritual beliefs, and none are necessarily right or wrong. What I have observed in my years in practice and in my own life, is that feeling connected spiritually profoundly impacts the way we see the world, including the way we view suffering. I have noticed that the people who are more spiritually connected are more able to feel grateful for their life, even in the face of their illness, and feel less hopeless about their disease. They feel less alone and take solace in their spiritual connection. Spiritual practices such as prayer and meditation are also very grounding and calming for the mind, which can lead to a reduction in pain and suffering.

People with strong faith also tend to adopt an outlook of serving others. I realize that this may sound paradoxical as many Lyme patients struggle even to get themselves the help they need, but I have noticed that those who reach out and help and support others, even if it is just a two-minute phone call to see how an elderly or another sick person is feeling, tend to be less hopeless about their own situation. Lyme patients are now uniquely positioned to have compassion and understanding for those who are still struggling.

REFERENCES

1. Strasheim C. 13 Lyme-literate practitioners share their healing strategies. 1st ed. Lake Tahoe: BioMed Publishing Group; 2009. 444 p.

2. Strasheim C. The Lyme disease survival guide: physical, lifestyle and emotional strategies for healing. 1st ed. Lake Tahoe: BioMed Publishing Group; 2008. 296 p.

3. Pert C. Molecules of emotion. 1st ed. Simon & Schuster; 1999. 368 p.

4. Doidge N. The brain that changes itself. 2nd ed. Penguin Books; 2008. 427 p.

21. STORIES OF HOPE AND RECOVERY

THERE ARE PEOPLE WITH LYME DISEASE WHO ARE RECOVERING, patients who have been through antibiotic treatment and are now off their medications and feeling well. There are many who have experienced significant improvement, and while not 100%, are back at work, living their lives, and functioning as they used to before they got sick.

Everyone's journey is different and everyone's concept of "better" or "recovered" is different. Some people will have to watch their nutrition closely. Others may still feel a flare up of fatigue when they are under stress, or will one day have to do medications again. No one is claiming that they will never deal with Lyme and its symptoms again. However, compared to what they suffered in the past, they are doing remarkably well. With a healthy diet, healthy lifestyle and healthy outlook, there is nothing to say that their recovery cannot be permanent.

I wanted to share some stories with you to show you this and encourage you along your recovery path. These are the stories of several of my patients both in the United States and overseas.

■ ■ ■ ■

Aimee S.

I grew up in a tick endemic area on the east coast of the United States. I had deer living in my yard, our cats have brought mice into the house, I trained for half marathons in the woods and I have even pulled ticks off of my husband after his mountain bike rides. I thought that I knew about Lyme disease as my immediate family members and friends had contracted it after being bitten by a tick and getting the hallmark EM rash. So you would think that when I came down with every single symptom on the symptom checklist for Lyme, Babesia and Bartonella, I would have said to myself, 'Hey, I think I have Lyme.' Well, I wish it were that simple. You see, I never recall being bitten by a tick or having a bull's eye rash, so the diagnosis of Lyme never crossed my mind. And so I began my journey of discovery and more importantly, healing.

After years of symptoms, I had finally talked my doctor into signing the paperwork and sending my blood off to IGeneX Labs. It is ironic because at this stage I was getting the tests done to rule out Lyme disease even though I thought it was a long shot. Although I did not have IGeneX test for Babesia or Bartonella, my tests came back IgM negative, but IgG positive, for Lyme. I had many positive and indeterminate bands present on both of these Lyme tests. From conducting my own research on how to read and understand IGeneX lab results, I realized that the numerous positive bands I did have meant that I most likely had Lyme. I decided to make an appointment with a LLMD who gave me a clinical diagnosis of Lyme, Babesia and Bartonella.

My Lyme treatment lasted a little over three years, and I was treated by two different doctors. My first LLMD was located in the States as I was living in America at the time. He prescribed antibiotics to target Lyme first and then the co-infections. He used high doses of one antibiotic at a time, and once I improved then plateau'd, I would move on to the next antibiotic on his schedule. I started with doxycycline, and then moved on to Zithromax, Ceftin, Flagyl and finally clindamycin & quinine. He also prescribed B-12 shots every other day, high doses of probiotics, magnesium, Diflucan for systematic yeast, Boulouke for biofilm and twice-daily injections of heparin for thinning out my blood so the bacteria couldn't hide in thick blood.

About a year into my treatment, my husband was transferred to Sydney, Australia for work. I tried coordinating overseas phone calls with my LLMD in order to continue my treatments, but it never worked. I was living in Australia with no doctor to treat me. About this time, I felt ready to change doctors because all of my research indicated that it is best to treat with multiple antibiotics concurrently rather than consecutively. I was also looking for a more holistic and integrated approach. That is when I found Dr. Nicola through one of the Australian Lyme Support Groups. By the time I had my first appointment with her, some of my symptoms had improved, but I was still struggling with crushing fatigue, severe brain fog, air hunger, insomnia, some anxiety and depression, and pain on the bottom of my feet. Since my first doctor and I hadn't really addressed co-infections yet, Dr. N and I felt strongly that they were causing most of my symptoms. Dr. N and I focused on treating Babesia and Bartonella as well as Lyme. While under Dr. N's care I was on a multiple-antibiotics approach and taking Flagyl, Zithromax, Biaxin, Mepron, and Lariam. It was with her antibiotic combination that I saw my symptoms disappear.

While my main form of treatment was antibiotics, I did rely heavily on other adjunct treatment modalities. About three months after being diagnosed I bought a Rife machine and used that to not only target Lyme and co-infections, but viruses as well. I do feel that my Rife machine was just as important as my antibiotics in terms of lowering my viral and bacterial load. Dr. N introduced me to colloidal silver, which I still use to this day. While killing the bugs is very important, detox was a top priority in my treatment protocol as well. Daily coffee enemas, Dr. N's herbal protocol, Dr. N's detox protocol, FIR sauna, Epsom salt baths, drinking three liters of lemon water a day, and lymphatic drainage massages were all used as part of my detox regime. After starting treatment with Dr. N, I began to see a chiropractor that knew about Lyme and we worked together to get my body realigned and functioning again. I believe this helped strengthen my immune system, provided relief from back & neck pain and gave me more flexibility and range of motion.

As part of my detox protocol I had to change my diet. I stopped eating gluten, wheat, soy, corn, starches, sugars and artificial sweeteners (I only use Stevia now). I have added more healthy fats such as coconut oil when cooking my meals. My new eating style is more aligned with a

Paleo, or primal, way of eating. Since making this change in my diet, I feel even better now than I did before I got sick with Lyme. I feel that cutting out these high allergy and inflammatory type foods has allowed my immune system to get stronger, and I have been healthier to fight Lyme and its co-infections.

The three years that I battled with Lyme were some of the toughest and darkest days I had ever experienced. Just getting out of bed in the morning seemed like a small victory at times. I knew that having Lyme was going to be the ultimate test of my own self-determination and resilience. I had decided early on to take the approach of healing not only from a physical aspect but from an emotional & spiritual one as well. So while I was using antibiotics, Rife, colloidal silver, herbals and detox protocols for the medical aspect, I was also treating the emotional and psychological aspects. I made the decision not to get 'stuck' in anger, resentment or sadness at how my life had changed, rather to look at my situation as a wake-up call or life lesson to be learned. I asked myself, 'How did I wind up in this predicament? Why did I get sick?' I don't believe that people just get Lyme for no reason. I believe that something in your body or in your lifestyle isn't healthy or working correctly and this allows you to get sick.

I am also a big believer that our thoughts and emotions are directly correlated to our state of health and wellbeing. I started seeing a therapist who specializes in Emotional Freedom Technique (EFT). This was a tremendous help and I was able to work through some of my mental blocks and negative self talk that I had been carrying around for years. I consider EFT instrumental in helping me get to where I am now. It also helped me realize that I when I was in remission from Lyme, I didn't want to go back to my old life, because that old lifestyle is what got me sick in the first place—high stress, poor eating habits, no sleep, always putting other people's needs before my own, and basically not taking care of myself. I had to put me first.

It is still a struggle to change, but I know if I want to stay in remission, it is what I have to do. I never thought I would say this, but I am glad I got sick with Lyme. It was my wakeup call that I had to change in order to keep myself healthy. I realized that Lyme was my body's way of telling me, 'Hey, we can't go on like this anymore. Something has to give.' I listened and responded to that wakeup call. I consider myself an even better, healthier person today than before I got sick.

I consider myself in remission as I have been off antibiotics for 1 ½ years. I continue to use colloidal silver and sometimes my Rife machine. In addition, I have added the salt and C protocol to my relapse prevention plan and it has kept me symptom free and living a full and active life for the past 1 ½ years. I only think about Lyme disease when I take my daily dose of salt and C. I do believe that remission is possible, but it has to be a multifaceted and holistic approach to healing. Now, when I make any life decisions, I ask, 'Is this in the best interest of my health?' I would have never thought this way three years ago.

■ ■ ■ ■

Jannine L.

When I was first tested for Lyme disease, it was through ELISA testing, which came back negative—shocker! The Western Blot only came back positive with an IgM and the doctors said it was a false positive. IGeneX was better and pulled more appropriate bands for Lyme. I was later tested for co-infections and came back positive for Babesia, however, with additional testing and experimenting with the Rife machine it was obvious I had Bartonella as well.

I started out treating with antibiotics—I believe doxycycline was the first. I was then cycled on three drugs at a time to go after all three forms. I was on antibiotics for a total of 1 1/2 years. I gave up antibiotics after realizing I was stagnant in my health and going nowhere. I felt that the antibiotics were doing more harm than good to my body at that time.

After stopping antibiotic treatment I underwent 60 dives at the HBOT clinic. It took about 3 months after treatment to finally feel the release and my first "I'm feeling better" feeling. I believe the delay was due to my body not being able to process all the toxins at the time. Hyperbarics got me up and going again—becoming more active, working out in the gym, with limitations, but slowly gaining back my life.

It was about one year post hyperbarics I could tell I was having regrowth of bugs but wanted to pursue another avenue. I came across the Doug coil rife machine. I coiled for one year straight focusing on Lyme, Bartonella, Babesia and Mycoplasma—and my life was finally turning around. I was able to go back to work and continued to chip away at the layers of these bugs one treatment at a time. I got to a point with coiling that I was having a hard time beating Bartonella while working and came upon a doctor Dr. Toby Watkinson who uses energy medicine and treats his patients with frequency-based remedies in a liquid form.

So the most helpful treatments for me have been the HBOT, the Doug coil machine and Dr. Toby's energy medicine. Through these I was also able to rebalance my thyroid, adrenals, pain, and detox within a very short time.

Nutrition also played a big role. I cannot say enough about nutrition - it is how we thrive. I adopted the Lyme inflammation diet mentioned in *The Lyme Disease Solution* by Ken Singleton.[1] I lived on this diet for a full year and it took my pain from a 9 to a 2 within 7 days. I would have not achieved that with just eating "healthy things" because some "healthy things" can still cause an individual pain. As my health and pain improved through removing bugs etc I can now eat pretty much anything, however from changing my diet initially I now crave large salads, homemade sauces and good quality foods. On a regular basis I avoid dairy and gluten. But I occasionally cheat and enjoy and do just fine.

Supplemental treatments and supports that helped me were RestorProbiotics, colonics (or coffee enemas if one can't afford colonics), and infrared saunas, which can be purchased inexpensively through Amazon. Welchol (a prescription medication used as a toxin binder) was by far the best detox agent for me. If I was Herxing from the Rife machine, a dose of Welchol on an empty stomach would calm it within a couple of hours.

In my case the antibiotics and herbal antimicrobials were the least helpful. If I were to start this journey all over again knowing what I know now I would do as above—buy a Rife machine and get a script for Welchol to help with the detox, see Dr. Toby for "re-balancing" and sit in my sauna.

It took me to this point almost 4 years of experimenting till I found the protocol that works best. I now tell/teach people what I have shared above. I am a firm believer that if you get the right coil machine (Doug coil) and if you can afford energy medicine such as Dr. Toby, you can be taking boot camp classes and living a healthy normal life in 2 years.

I am not a religious person so I did not draw on faith in God per se, but I did though tell myself on hard days that "I was happy to be alive, tomorrow will be better, people have it worse than me etc". This pep talk always helped to remind me that it could be worse. I found it okay to cry out loud on the days where that was needed—it felt good afterwards, like a nice relief; chatting with other Lyme victims always helped as well.

My plans on staying well include:

1. Nutrition – I will continue to eat well and thrive well. Even when I feel great and cheat and start eating a lot of "non veggies" I find that my body just loves better nutrition. In addition, the more people I speak with who are older than me and non-diseased have said that nutrition has kept them healthier, leaner, more energetic and overall happier. We can never downplay nutrition!

2. Exercise – I now do boot camp three times a week, slave in my yard and walk my dogs daily. "The body will keep moving till you're 100 if you keep making it."

3. Living in a dryer climate if possible.

4. Handle stress more appropriately. Stress was my initial downfall that opened "Pandora's box of hell." People have no idea how it takes a toll on the immune system and how disease can take a hold when the body is weakened by stress.

5. Use my rife machine for any other viruses/bacteria my body comes in contact with over the years. I will never part with that machine.

6. Be happy that I'm healthy and living a normal life and continue to help others shorten their journey!!

■ ■ ■ ■

Len F.

I am Len, now from San Diego, CA previously from Middletown/Red Bank area of NJ. I was definitely infected in New Jersey (NJ). My story starts out the same as many of you chronically affected Lyme patients; I was infected back in 1990 and misdiagnosed for 10 years allowing the disease to become chronic. During that time I was treated for depression and the flu while constantly being told by various doctors that my symptoms sound like Lyme disease but all those blood tests never confirmed Lyme disease. Of course, other doctors stated there was nothing wrong with me when in fact I suffered from chronic neurological Lyme disease.

Here is a list of the symptoms I was experiencing:

- Light-headedness, wooziness, sometimes needing to sit or lie
- Weather related—high outside temperatures usually worsen the above [maybe direct sun]
- Off balance
- Vision issues
- Eyes painful, light sensitivity
- Severe headaches—migraines & stabbing side headaches
- Confusion and difficulty concentrating- too painful
- Word search & name block
- Forgetfulness, poor attention
- Brain fog
- Sound sensitivity
- Ears buzzing, ringing & hurting - mostly right side
- Flu symptoms from time to time—mostly during Herx—running nose, etc.
- Motion sickness
- Nausea
- Queasy stomach with gas
- Pain in the lower right abdomen area above where the appendix was
- Sore throat
- Breathlessness, air hunger, unexplained chronic cough
- Coughing/swallowing at the same result in spitting food out

- Depression
- Avoiding people or talking to people
- Neck pain—head too heavy for the neck; creaks, cracks, and stiff-ness
- Lower back pain and right hip pains
- All joints in the body ache at the same time - worse in am
- Sore ankles and heel of foot - worse in am
- Leg twitching when lying down
- Electricity traveling up/down my arms from the shoulder to wrist
- Numbness in arms and hands, especially left arm and right hand
- Numbness in hands & foot
- Leg/calf cramping
- Spots on leg just start to hurt then rotate elsewhere
- Spots on leg that are very sensitive to the touch
- Isolated pains that move around the body
- Chest wall pain, sore ribs, heart pain & pressure
- Under left arm pit gland swelling from a tick that was embedded there for over 30 days
- Itching that moves around the body
- Feeling the start of Bell's palsy on left side of face at times or start of a stroke
- Herpes I and II
- Pain in the genital area
- Erratic bowel movements—from diarrhea to constipation
- Chronic fatigue
- Sleeping problems—usually wake up every 2-3 hours
- Napping during the day due to being tired or fatigue, sometimes weak
- Some night sweats
- Chills changing to hot most of the time

Finally, in November 2000, I finally came up positive on a blood test for Lyme disease and I immediately contacted a Lyme-literate doctor in New Jersey who immediately ordered an IGeneX lab set of blood tests and placed me on doxycycline. The New Jersey doctor's blood test from

IGeneX labs did confirm Lyme disease, but I was never told that 2000 test also indicated Babesia and Ehrlichia.

I was treated for the next 8 years with various antibiotics and supplements and lived a roller coaster life, from being very sick to short periods of betterment. Since I now lived in San Diego I decided to switch doctors from a NJ doctor to a local Lyme-literate doctor (the author of this book) in April 2009.

What a miracle.

Dr. M switched my meds to Mepron, Azithromycin, Alinia, and at times Rifampin, along with various supplements and was able to bring be back from bed ridden considering suicide (as I had no quality of life) to 70% of my normal life. Just about when I had lost hope a savior came along.

I continued with Dr. M utilizing her treatment of antibiotics coupled with naturopathic support until September 2009 when I learned from the Lyme video entitled "Under Our Skin" of a doctor in upstate NY who appeared to be one of the remaining experts now that Dr. Burrascano had closed his practice. So I decided to switch, which became an expensive mistake.

The NY doctor managed to take me from 70% of normal health down to 10%. Again, I became desperate, as my quality of life was horrible, so I returned to Dr. M to help.

Once again, Dr. M utilized her cocktail and had me improving within 3 months and back to 70% within 6 months; that is right from 10% to 70% in 6 months—another miracle.

Today, I have enjoyed 90% of normal for approximately 1 1/2 years and hope it continues. However, to stay well I still take antibiotics and supplements, and may need to do so indefinitely. Currently I am taking:

- Malarone
- Alinia
- Bactrim DS
- Doxycycline

- Azithromycin

I also take thyroid medication as my thyroid function is low, another impact of this disease.

My current supplements include probiotics (two different kinds), liver support, NAC, grapefruit seed extract (for yeast and cyst forms of Borrelia), fish oil, ashwaghanda (for adrenal support), B complex, Vitamin C, Soothe and Relaxx (containing magnesium and herbal anti-inflammatories) and Vitamin D.

Here are some of the lessons I learned that might be helpful in your journey:

1. My labs never matched my clinical diagnosis so be careful. As a matter of fact, while I was on antibiotics the lab results were often inaccurate. I only trust IGeneX lab results.

2. Since I never reviewed or understood my own lab results in 2000, I did not know that I was only being treated for Lyme and not the co-infections. In my opinion, recovery depends on Babesia being treated first or in conjunction with Lyme and the other co-infections.

3. Without a bundled antibiotic and naturopathic treatment you will not stay well. Contrary to what some other doctors are saying, I do not believe that 100% naturopathic treatment will return a chronically infected Lyme patient back to any significant level of normalcy, but naturopathic treatment is an important addition to the antibiotic treatment. Forget the miracle cures from various web sites and doctors, the ones I tried only made me worse.

4. While you are severely ill your faith will be challenged. Please know that "mostly better" does exist and find the right doctor and cocktail. PLEASE HANG IN THERE.

In closing, I just want to assure you there is hope and betterment out there. You need to continue the fight until you locate the correct doctor and the proper cocktail.

■ ■ ■ ■

Rhonda M.

I was finally diagnosed with Lyme disease in April 2008 after returning from Scotland and Bavaria and being sick for four years. During this time I was diagnosed with a range of illnesses from meningitis and Bell's palsy to severe ongoing headaches, muscle weakness, extreme fatigue, depression, skin and bowel disorders, to name a few. Each of the diagnoses had been individually treated. At this time I was put on doxycycline for three weeks. As I was not improving I had a lumbar puncture done which confirmed the disease was in my central nervous system, and then received 30 days of 2g intravenous ceftriaxone, after which a second lumbar puncture was done and came back negative for the infection.

Once the IV treatment started my symptoms increased to include speech and reading difficulties, and problems performing normal activities to the extent at times it became dangerous (e.g. pouring water into the electrical component of the bread maker and not the bowl). I found these mental difficulties to be very unsettling as I had gone from running professional development in curriculum development for teachers; along with parent information sessions; and modeling and mentoring colleagues in best teaching practice, to being unable to put sentences together correctly at times, and unable to read, to the extent that I felt like a child learning to read. My specialist could not explain this and put it down to Chronic Fatigue and Fibromyalgia, but my symptoms were constantly changing. What I experienced one day might not be what happened the next! I was referred to a neurologist who couldn't find anything during a physical examination but was going to access my history next time he was in the hospital. I never heard from him again.

As Lyme disease is not found in Australia (or so I was told at the time), it was difficult to get answers. My infectious disease specialist had seen very few cases of Lyme and had not treated someone who had been infected for four years. He told me that I had been given the best treatment possible (he kept referring to a little book from Stanford University, obviously the IDSA treatment guidelines) and that hopefully by Christmas, I would have more good days than bad. I started to improve and then would go backwards. It was difficult because I was not sure what to expect, and there was no one to really discuss it with.

I consulted an integrative medicine physician who found I was deficient in a number of vitamins and minerals. I had seven weekly IV treatments with Vitamin B, eight with vitamin C and zinc, and two with magnesium. I also took supplements for all of these except Vitamin C. This doctor picked up that I had a thyroid problem, as I had high thyroid antibodies and started treating me with thyroid medication.

Fortunately one of the nurses who had been treating me while I was having intravenous treatment visited Germany for a holiday and spoke to a friend about Lyme disease treatment in Germany. She returned to Australia and contacted me with the website details for the Borreliose Centrum Augsburg (BCA) in Augsburg, suggesting it would be worth contacting them to see if they could offer any advice on this disease.

After waiting a few months I was at my wits end and so one night, I emailed BCA. My husband thought that they wouldn't reply or would tell me to go to Germany. To our surprise we received a response the next morning from one of the doctors at BCA, saying I had not had the best treatment with oral antibiotics, and that the IV treatment was insufficient in both dose and the amount of time given. I was also told that after four years I had chronic Lyme disease. He suggested that I needed to be tested for co-infections and, "The first step for you is looking for Lyme activity in your blood by Elispot-LTT and CD-57 count." He also told me what treatment I needed and was happy to speak to my specialist, and so began my long journey towards recovery.

My infectious disease specialist started the new regimen of IV ceftriaxone at the increased dose, which was pulsed at four days on/ three days off each week, with weekly blood tests done here. He didn't think it was necessary to have the blood tested by the clinic in Germany, however after discussions with the doctor at BCA, we decided to send the blood sample to Germany. This was the best decision we could have made since the results came back showing both Lyme disease and Chlamydia pneumonia. I had IV treatment for nine weeks, and initially my specialist was supportive. However, as the weeks passed and I was admitted to the hospital a couple of times, he began to change his attitude and say that it was "all in my head." The clinic in Germany had sent articles regarding Lyme and co-infections and the necessary treatment, which we passed on to the specialist. When asked at one of the weekly consultations whether he had read the articles, his response was, "No, I don't have time." I found these weekly consultations to be very distressing but was always supported by the fantastic nurses from "Hospital in The Home" who were caring for me and the doctor from BCA, with whom I had regular contact and who would respond quickly to any concerns.

At the beginning of week eight I again sent blood to Germany, and my specialist had decided he was going to stop IV treatment straight away. We managed to persuade him to continue until the results came back a few days later. These indicated that I still had both infections but the Chlamydia needed to be treated. I changed to Phase 2 of treatment as recommended by BCA, which involved oral antibiotics—clarithromycin and Plaquenil for 12 weeks, fortnightly blood tests for liver, kidney and blood count and sending blood to Germany every eight weeks. By this stage I had experienced enough of the negative attitude of the specialist impacting negatively on my health, and after discussion with my local doctor, decided that I would be better off having him supervise my care. He has been fantastic and even organized for my blood to be taken at the clinic and transported to BCA. He could see that I still required treatment but believed that I should not have to go overseas to be treated. BCA's protocol involved having a break for four weeks and then sending blood again. After this I began Phase 3 of treatment. The oral antibiotics changed to azithromycin which was again a pulsed therapy and Plaquenil for 12 weeks, and we continued to send blood for testing.

In October 2009 after 12 months of antibiotic treatment, BCA recommended I go off all antibiotics for another 12 weeks and build up my immune system (the latest results still indicated that I had a very high cellular active Chlamydia pneumonia infection and a high cellular Lyme infection. I also had symptoms for a Bartonella-like organism co-infection). While I was happy to be off the antibiotics, I was very concerned and distressed about the possibility of the infections getting worse again.

After further discussion with BCA, I pointed out that right from the start, I had been building up my immune system as they had advised with the help of an integrative doctor, I and I couldn't see how I would improve without some sort of additional support over the next 12 weeks. I was really concerned that I wouldn't be able to function and would end back where I started. After much discussion and review of my symptoms, it was recommended that I change to an herbal and naturopathic pathway.

This presented a problem for me as the medical system in Australia does not promote naturopathic therapies as is the case in Europe. In general our medical system does not practice "holistic" medicine, which is what I needed. BCA offered to send me the name and contact number of someone who could do phone consultations with my practitioner in Australia. At this stage and after having read Dr. Whitmont's article in the book, *Insights Into Lyme Disease Treatment* by Connie Strasheim, I found a medically trained classical homeopath who had some experience in treating Lyme started homeopathic treatment. This homeopath was very caring and after doing some research recommended that I try Rife treatment via an F-Scan compact machine, which he ordered so he could treat me. I was responding and showing signs of improvement. It was then Christmas, and he loaned me the machine to use every second day while the clinic was closed, and then he continued the treatment himself. It was at this stage that I deteriorated rapidly and ended up worse than I had ever been. The homeopath recommended that I needed to see my doctor to determine the next steps. My doctor was still more than happy to support me in my treatment but wanted to be guided by someone who had considerable experience in treating Lyme disease. It was agreed that I would contact Dr. Nicola.

I was too ill to do anything so my husband sent an email to Dr. Nicola at the end of January 2010 and within two days we had scheduled a phone consultation. This was the beginning of many long distance consultations via the phone and Skype. I was also fortunate enough to be able to see Dr. Nicola in Sydney and Canberra. Dr. Nicola gradually introduced antibiotic, herbal and naturopathic supplements, which continued until January 2011. This treatment focused on Lyme, Babesia and Bartonella and was quite difficult at times. Apart from the Herxing, which I experienced, I also had a severe reaction to Alinia, which took me a couple of weeks to get over with the help of my osteopath and massage therapist (all my muscles had been adversely affected and I struggled to move). It was very much a case of working out which antibiotics worked for me. Progress was slow and seemed to be one step forward two steps back, but Dr. Nicola kept reassuring me that I would come through this, and that there was light at the end of the tunnel. The doctor at BCA had also said it was a very long process and that "patients needed to be patient." I would often think that I wasn't making much progress only to suddenly realize that I was able to do something again that I hadn't been able to do several months before. BCA had encouraged me to keep a record of symptoms, which was very helpful in recognizing the changes in both symptoms and severity; when you are feeling so ill, it is easy to forget so you may not notice subtle changes.

In January 2011 I looked at the possibility of going off antibiotics and returning to the naturopathic pathway. My doctor was concerned that I would regress after coming so far. At this stage it felt right to me, and I could always go back on antibiotics. After discussion with Dr. Nicola, we decided I would start coming off antibiotics one at a time and very slowly so we could monitor what was happening. These antibiotics were replaced with olive leaf and colloidal silver but I continued to use all the other supplements from Dr. Nicola. I was feeling quite well but would still experience setbacks.

Through the BCA I learned about the importance of a holistic approach to treatment. I needed to support my recovery on many levels, as I was about to experience a roller coaster ride. They encouraged me to download the Burrascano guidelines, which I was able to give to my doctors, and to purchase Dr. Kenneth Singleton's book *The Lyme Disease Solution*. These became constant resources along with BCA's website and Connie Strasheim's book *Insights Into Lyme Disease Treatment*.

As part of the holistic approach to regaining my health, I built up a team of supporting professionals to work alongside me in my journey, some of whom I had worked with prior to my diagnosis. Alongside BCA, Dr.

Nicola and my local doctor, these people helped to play a crucial role in helping me through extremely difficult times to regain my health.

I was fortunate enough to have the support of a psychologist who I had worked with while teaching. Being told that I had nothing wrong with me and needed to have counseling was very draining and set me back emotionally. The psychologist gave me strategies to deal with this set-back and support to deal with the chronic illness and resulting depression. He offered strategies to ensure that my husband and I always had the appropriate support.

My osteopath took the time to research Lyme disease after I was diagnosed. He utilized a number of treatments over the years and I responded very well to Biodynamic Cranial Osteopathy. The osteopath said, "as the infection gets into all parts of your body, the biggest benefit is that this treatment helps your whole body work together to heal all of its parts and as such, all parts benefit from the treatment. It especially helps your neuro-endocrine-immune system work as a whole to fight the infection." He also worked closely with my massage therapist and myotherapist. He discussed my personal needs with my personal trainer and Pilates instructor, both of whom had been given the ILADS information about physical activity and its role in healing. It didn't matter how bad I was feeling, they encouraged me to attend my sessions and would adapt them accordingly, many times just gently getting my muscles moving. They also believed that getting me out of the house, even for a short time, would assist my general well-being.

Despite using several sleep remedies, sleep remained a major issue in my recovery. I was lucky to have one hour of sleep a night, and everyone was concerned about the impact on my body healing. At times I had to resort to strong sleep medication. As a result I tried hypnotherapy and acupuncture without success. I eventually came across Ondamed therapy, which is a form of energy medicine, and while reluctant and skeptical about this I was eventually desperate enough to give it a go. This was to become a core part of my treatment program because it addressed both my sleep and other health issues. I also used other treatments such as far-infra red sauna and Epson salt baths to assist with detox, aromatherapy and meditation.

Diet played a major role in my treatment and helped to reduce toxins and inflammation throughout my body. Just prior to my Lyme diagnosis I was diagnosed with fructose malabsorption, gluten intolerance and lactose intolerance, and as a result, my diet changed to gluten free. The BCA clinic recommended a Mediterranean diet as it was anti-inflammatory. This required some adjustments due to the fructose malabsorption issues but was easily managed as long I watched the type and quantity of fruit I was eating at one time. Adjusting my diet has made a big difference to my general well-being.

My personal faith through prayer and meditation has been vital in coping with the illness. It was comforting to know that others within the faith communities were also praying for me.

From the time of diagnosis it has taken about 3 1/2 years to start feeling well enough to be able to participate more fully in everyday activities. Improvement was gradual and I would often suddenly realize I was able to do things I hadn't been able to do in a long time. The day I was able to start reading again and not feel like a child learning to read was truly wonderful. Being able to walk up and down stairs at a relative's home was another great step forward, quickly followed by realizing that I could go for walks again no matter how small to start with. It was important to remember not to overdo things because I was feeling good that day, and even now, I try to follow the advice of my psychologist to only do 70% of what I feel I can do comfortably, and then have a break and go back to it. Of course, sometimes, I forget these wise words, and when I do, I always feel worse after pushing myself.

Last year I was able to travel through outback Australia for 13 weeks and coped very well. We did as much planning as possible to ensure things went smoothly for me, including buying a caravan that had an en-suite for the days when it would be too much for me to walk to the amenity block at the caravan park. I worked with my local doctor to ensure that I had enough medication plus a back-up plan for an emergency (which wasn't needed but was great to have). We also worked out how far I could comfortably travel within a day without getting tired, and we had a healthy diet of fresh and home-cooked food. This was a great experience and really lifted my spirits, helping me to feel like my old self again. We now go away once a month for a weekend with the caravan club, something I look forward to. As a rule, when we go out of a night, we don't stay out late, which gives me the best possible chance of staying well. This also means that I can participate in more social activities.

I don't know if I will ever fully recover. I still experience setbacks but these generally only last a day or two. Today I would consider myself to be somewhere around 90% recovered. But I believe it is important to remember that I have also gotten older and there are some natural aging changes. I find it helpful to think of the Lyme bacteria in the following way (pointed out to me by my local naturopath/homeopath): "Once you have had chicken pox, the bacteria stay in your body but your body is able to live in harmony with it for most of the time. Lyme bacteria could be the same as it may not be possible to eradicate every single bacteria." I am now more vigilant about my health and have learned to listen to my body and respond to its needs rather than pushing myself to keep going and meet other's demands.

Today I try to improve my current state of health by building and supporting my immune, adrenal and nervous systems, through the advice and support of a local Naturopath/Homeopath, Osteopath, Myotherapist, Ondamed therapist, Pilates instructor, Personal Trainer, regular meditation and diet as well as detoxing.

For those suffering with Lyme, don't give up hope of ever regaining your health. Be aware that lab results may not match your diagnosis. Fortunately my initial lab results showed Lyme infection, otherwise I would have never been diagnosed. However they didn't show the extent of the infection or the co-infections. If doctors tell you to stop treatment, check with and be guided by doctors experienced in treating Lyme who work with symptoms. Be gentle on yourself and take things slowly. Do not take medical advice as gospel, which I naively did in the early days. Be proactive in your treatment and listen to your body. You will know what is right for you.

■ ■ ■ ■

Marisa F.

I was bitten in Mazatlan, Mexico in 2009 while on a cruise. It was an insect that bit me while I was in the water, but I am uncertain exactly what it was. After that I had some lesions on my leg but they faded and I felt ok. About a month later, I started feeling ill. I had been doing a lot of gardening at my home in San Diego, but do not recall another bite.

The doctors I saw did not have a lot information about Lyme and it was me who had to do most of the research and went to get myself a lab test for Lyme. The labs did show that I was positive for Lyme—at least then I had a clear diagnosis.

It took me 5 months to look for a doctor who specialized in Lyme disease. In those months, not only did I lose time, I was treated incorrectly with steroids (which are detrimental for Lyme patients) and developed arthritis. I was also not checked for co-infections at that time and only later found out I had Babesia.

I took antibiotics for Lyme and Babesia for almost two years. I took everything orally. To detox my body, I took a variety of antimicrobial herbal formulas and for my Lyme and Babesia, I took vitamin supplements, dietary supplements, iron, acidophilus, adrenal support, thyroid and sexual hormones, cortisol, analgesics and soft tissue and stress support.

Even though I have always eaten healthfully, my diet eventually changed to gluten free and lactose free because it made a big difference in my arthritis and skin problems. Also, when I was on antibiotics, it was extremely important not to eat too much fat and avoid feeling nauseated.

Antibiotics for Lyme and Babesia and Mepron treatment for Babesia were definitely the most helpful. I was concerned with my liver because it showed high toxicity but using the herbal detox formula and glutathione helped it a lot and I was able to continue my medications.

The least helpful thing was taking Ibuprofen when I had a lot of pain in my swollen ankle. Honestly, I did not feel it took my pain away and only gave me gastritis. Also, the analgesics did not work for my constant headaches. When my skin lesions were really severe, nothing that I took or used topically helped me besides antibiotics.

When I realized that Herxheimer reaction meant that I was destroying the Lyme bacteria itself, I was sometimes scared and overwhelmed. Although it made me feel very sick and my brain very foggy, I felt that was a good thing and something good was about to happen out of all this. I started recovering slowly. It is extremely important to keep a journal of your signs and symptoms, and to keep track of doctor's appointments and medications.

In the beginning I did not pay too much attention to how long it takes to get better when you have Lyme and Babesia. I thought that treatment was going to be just a few months but as time passed I became very desperate. When I read that a patient has to be asymptomatic for at least 4 months to discontinue antibiotics, I decided to keep a journal which helped me to realize not to have false expectations and that my medical treatment would stop soon.

If I could do something differently in hindsight it would be to read more about this disease and understand the importance of both rest and diet (gluten and dairy free) for recovery.

Something that I experienced and I can suggest for you is to not let people pressure you (even your own family who loves you) with comments insinuating that the disease is taking too long to treat, that nothing is working, you are taking to many antibiotics and for so long, too many side effects, and to look for more medical opinions. This is when my symptom journal helped me because I was keeping track of how I felt, always remembering that 4 months had to pass by symptom free.

The psycho-emotional aspects of the disease were tough. I never got professional psychological help. Also I could not lean much on friends or family because at that time also my father was sick, so I gave myself the only therapy that I could figure out. I went for walks and cheered myself up to continue taking medications and to handle the side effects as well my skin problems that they where very painful, itchy and drove me sometimes crazy. While having insomnia I read and watched videos on You Tube about Lyme and they were the same or worse than me, and

I thanked God I was going much better and it was only another relapse and it will go eventually away in few days.

I got very little support from my family because I live by myself with my two daughters. When you are the sole breadwinner of your house and you see how much your kids depend economically and physically on you, somewhere you find the strength to try to be well as soon as possible and continue working any way you can. It is tough to afford medical insurance and pay all your bills.

It was hard for family to see that you feel sick and very tired but really don't understand, you because even for you all this is something new that is changing your way of living very much. Those days that everything hurts and you can not believe that you live in that body at night trying to go to sleep or waking up in the morning after having a terrible night with pain and insomnia, you thank God for not being worse – perhaps not being able to walk or having seizures or mental problems. When I watched videos and went to a support group of Lyme victims, I realized that I was not as bad as many, and all I needed to do was keep taking my medications, eat well and rest as much as possible.

It took me 2 years to be symptom free of Lyme and Babesia, but while those symptoms and skin problems were going away I started being extremely tired, waking up feeling like a battery that would not recharge and at noon feel like it was 2am. I was extremely tired and with no desire to exercise and very sleepy throughout the day. Fortunately I was diagnosed with hormonal imbalance (mainly cortisol) so with adrenal support treatment, I have been feeling again much better. I was afraid that my Lyme symptoms were coming back, but at that point it was more the effects of chronic illness of my body that I had to address, not the infection itself.

My major plans to stay well are to eat healthy, exercise but listen to my body and rest as much I can.

■ ■ ■ ■

Fiona B.

One of the first things people ask me when they discover that I have Lyme disease is, "How long have you had it?" My answer is simply that I have no idea. I have been unwell for many years but had plenty of justifications for all the symptoms individually, and I guess I also suffered from martyrdom and I just got on with it. It wasn't until I really couldn't stay awake after lunchtime, was in unbearable physical pain, vomited daily, had distortions with my vision and a brain that seem to find basic functioning hard that I sought medical advice. I fortunately have a general practitioner that took it seriously. After months and months of testing and eliminating lots of different possibilities, I got a CD-57 test result that allowed my doctor to confidently but unofficially diagnose Lyme disease and immediately start me on an antibiotic program. Not long after this I was introduced to Dr. Nicola and as luck would have it my doctor was very willing to work with her. For the next 18 months I trusted my treatment program entirely to those two. For the most part I took between three and five different antibiotics daily, and numerous naturopathic remedies to support it. I did do some IGeneX testing which came back unable to deny or confirm the diagnosis. Fortunately my doctor wasn't swayed by this at all and continued supporting this intensive treatment plan.

One of the hardest parts of this medical/naturopathic plan for me was trying to manage and understand it. My brain didn't work so well and there was a complex concoction of dosing combinations! I focused on just trying to get the right doses on the right dates and happily left the planning to my medical team. To this day I am not entirely sure which drugs and herbs I took and when. Some people find this odd, but for me it was all just too much information that I couldn't manage. My Lyme disease story actually highlights that I compartmentalized it into areas that I needed to take responsibility for, and areas I could trust to others. I was happy with my medical team taking the responsibility for the treatment plan.

I did some research into the disease early on, which was necessary for me to get a sense of how serious this was. I needed some perspective. The next natural step for me was to grieve. I felt a real anger at the world and a sense of sadness at the loss of my life. I made contact with the Lyme community and read everything I could. After a while, this became counter-productive. I felt overwhelmed and ultimately despairing. It seemed such a hopeless situation and I struggled to find any positives.

I guess this is when my recovery changed for me. I asked myself, "If this is as good as it is going to get, then what could I be grateful for today?" So I began to put into practice what I as a coach helped other people do. I started to work on the mind, body, spirit approach to my disease.

Body - I looked at my diet and while far from perfect, I tried to eliminate food and drinks that didn't work. I cut out gluten, dairy, sugar and yeast. I ensured my vitamin and mineral intake was sufficient. I aimed to do a little bit of exercise every week to keep my body moving. Ten minutes walking was sometime my limit, but I committed to doing it. I allowed myself to sleep when I needed to and began listening to my body as to when to push a bit and when to rest.

Mind - This was the area in which I had the most control and also the area that not only assisted in feeling better, but made my journey to recovery easier emotionally. I did not want to stay in the place of being angry, overwhelmed and despairing, so I stopped fighting and started to accept that I had Lyme. I chose to focus on how I could maintain a positive attitude even if I felt terrible. I looked at what was still good, I made gratitude lists, I stopped feeling sorry for myself and took interest in other people, and I focused on what was good in my life, even if it was hard to find. Some days this was so hard when I felt so ill, and so sometimes I allowed myself to have a poor mental attitude day, knowing that this day would pass, and tomorrow I could be positive again. I also stopped believing that my fate would be the same as all the people talking to each other in the online communities. I started to know that I would recover and planned for the things that I would do as evidence of it. I watched people run up a hill and planned to cycle up it when I was well again. Daily I gave myself a pat on the back for a job well done! The actions I took regarding my mind were numerous but the intention was simply to cleanse my mind of toxins.

Spirit - Fortunately for me I had developed a faith in a higher power in the last decade, and I turned to that during this period. I trusted that all would be fine, that it would all work out OK, and that I was being looked after. My spirituality is a personal experience and impossible to describe, but it was important for me to have this connection throughout.

After about 16 months of antibiotic treatment, I finally took my last tablet. I still had symptoms and felt unwell but I had a strong sense of knowing that the symptoms that persisted were not Lyme. I knew it was different. Five months later I am still off antibiotics and getting stronger daily. I have had to deal with other issues and am not 100%, but the comparison between now and last year is strikingly different.

I do not know if I have recovered from Lyme, am in remission, or what. All I know is that for the last few months I have begun functioning again. I am beginning to re-engage with life, and my biggest fear is losing it all again and going back into that dark, deep hole of two years ago. My journey of recovery will be life long. I need to continue doing all things that are good for my mind, body and spirit. I choose to remain positive, to enjoy each day, to set goals for the future and to keep perspective. Not every headache is an indicator that I am relapsing! I am still working on the goal of cycling up a hill and yet I know I will do it.

Given the opportunity again, I am not sure I would do anything differently. In a strange way I am grateful for my experience. My hope for my future though is that experiencing this once is enough in this lifetime!

REFERENCES

1. Singleton K. The Lyme disease solution. 1st. ed. Charleston: BookSurge Publishing; 2009. 550 p.

CONCLUSION

WE HAVE COVERED A LOT OF GROUND IN THIS BOOK, BUT THERE is a lot of ground to be covered. That is the nature of Lyme disease.

Chronic Lyme disease is a very real, very serious illness. It has unique complexities and multiple facets that must be understood. Governments and health authorities have restricted knowledge and information about it, making it one of the most politicized illnesses of all time, and at the same time making accurate testing and treatment difficult for patients to obtain.

But let us not harp on that. The focus now needs to be changing the situation and getting accurate and appropriate recognition of Lyme disease. That in turn will translate to accurate and appropriate care for people affected by it.

Success in that area is dependent on raising awareness, supporting research efforts, and generating funding. Education of health practitioners is necessary so that they know what to look out for, and so that they consider Lyme disease as a diagnosis.

Internationally, ILADS is at the forefront of the promotion and education of doctors worldwide. They have email groups, physician training programs, annual conferences and treatment guidelines, all of which are available to doctors worldwide.

Change is coming. In fact, change is already here. It might be slower than we would hope, and it might not originate from the sources we have traditionally trusted to give us accurate information about our health and the threats to our health, but thanks to the courage of the many Lyme disease sufferers who have spoken out, the tenacity of those who have seen their loved ones suffer and who are determined to make a difference, the curiosity of the media, and the truth, which ultimately always wins out, Lyme disease is gaining recognition as a recognized disease. As time goes on, treatment options will expand, doctors will be trained, and many more people will have their own stories of hope and recovery to share.

APPENDICES

APPENDIX A

Burrascano's Treatment Guidelines 2008

ADVANCED TOPICS IN LYME DISEASE

DIAGNOSTIC HINTS AND TREATMENT GUIDELINES FOR LYME AND OTHER TICK BORNE ILLNESSES

Sixteenth Edition
Copyright October, 2008

JOSEPH J. BURRASCANO JR., M.D.

Board Member,
International Lyme and Associated
Diseases Society

TABLE OF CONTENTS

Welcome to the sixteenth edition of the "Guidelines".
Amazingly, this edition is not only the sixteenth in the series, but as the first edition appeared in 1984, this reflects *twenty four years of effort!*

New information is constantly being uncovered, and my goal is to keep this monograph as current as possible. Very recently, increased sharing of information among practitioners who care for people with chronic conditions such as Lyme, CFIDS, autism, Gulf War syndrome, chronic toxin exposure, autoimmune diseases of unknown origin, and others marks the dawning of a new age of medical enlightenment. Unfortunately, the huge quantity of information that embodies these separate but related conditions makes it ever more difficult for any one practitioner to 'do it all". This current edition, admittedly a work in progress as I try to assemble this new data, is the beginning of my effort to incorporate some relevant information learned from my work in these other fields, in an effort to better diagnose and treat those who have become ill, especially those who are chronically ill, as a result of exposure to tick-borne diseases.

I once again extend my best wishes to the many Lyme patients and their caregivers whose wisdom I deeply appreciate, and a sincere thank you to my colleagues whose endless contributions have helped me shape my approach to tick borne illnesses. I hope that this new edition proves to be useful. Happy reading!

BACKGROUND INFORMATION

WHAT IS LYME DISEASE?
I take a broad view of what Lyme Disease actually is. Traditionally, Lyme is defined an infectious illness caused by the spirochete, *Borrelia burgdorferi* (Bb). While this is certainly technically correct, clinically the illness often is much more than that, especially in the disseminated and chronic forms.

Instead, I think of Lyme as the illness that results from the bite of an infected tick. This includes infection not only with *B. burgdorferi*, but the many co-infections that may also result. Furthermore, in the chronic form of Lyme, other factors can take on an ever more significant role- immune dysfunction, opportunistic infections, co-infections, biological toxins, metabolic and hormonal imbalances, deconditioning, etc. I will refer to infection with *B. burgdorferi* as "Lyme Borreliosis" (LB), and use the designation "Lyme" and "Lyme Disease" to refer to the more broad definition I described above.

GENERAL PRINCIPLES
In general, you can think of LB as having three categories: acute, early disseminated, and chronic. The sooner treatment is begun after the start of the infection, the higher the success rate. However, since it is easiest to cure early disease, this category of LB must be taken VERY seriously. Undertreated infections will inevitably resurface, usually as chronic Lyme, with its tremendous problems of morbidity and difficulty with diagnosis and treatment and high cost in every sense of the word. So, while the bulk of this document focuses of the more problematic chronic patient, strong emphasis is also placed on earlier stages of this illness where closest attention and care must be made.

A very important issue is the definition of **"Chronic Lyme Disease"**. Based on my clinical data and the latest published information, I offer the following definition. To be said to have chronic LB, these three criteria must be present:
1. Illness present for at least one year (this is approximately when immune breakdown attains clinically significant levels).
2. Have persistent major neurologic involvement (such as encephalitis/encephalopathy, meningitis, etc.) or active arthritic manifestations (active synovitis).
3. Still have active infection with B. burgdorferi (Bb), regardless of prior antibiotic therapy (if any).

Chronic Lyme is an altogether different illness than earlier stages, mainly because of the inhibitory effect on the immune system (Bb has been demonstrated *in vitro* to both inhibit and kill B- and T-cells, and will decrease the count of the CD-57 subset of the natural killer cells). As a result, not only is the infection with Bb perpetuated and allowed to advance, but the entire issue of co-infections arises. Ticks may contain and transmit to the host a multitude of potential pathogens. The clinical presentation of Lyme therefore reflects which pathogens are present and in what proportion. Apparently, in early infections, before extensive damage to the immune system has occurred, if the germ load of the co-infectors is low, and the Lyme is treated, many of the other tick-transmitted microbes can be contained and eliminated by the immune system. However, in the chronic patient, because of the inhibited defenses, the individual components of the co-infection are now active enough so that they too add to features of the illness and must be treated. In addition, many latent infections which may have pre-dated the tick bite, for example herpes viruses, can reactivate, thus adding to the illness.

An unfortunate corollary is that serologic tests can become *less* sensitive as the infections progress, obviously because of the decreased immune response upon which these tests are based. In addition, immune complexes form, trapping Bb antibodies. These complexed antibodies are not detected by serologic testing. Not surprisingly the seronegative patient will convert to seropositive 36% of the time after antibiotic treatment has begun and a recovery is underway. Similarly, the antibody titer may rise, and the number of bands on the western blot may increase as treatment progresses and the patient recovers. Only years after a successfully treated infection will the serologic response begin to diminish.

The severity of the clinical illness is directly proportional to the spirochete load, the duration of infection, and the presence of co-infections. These factors also are proportional to the intensity and duration of treatment needed for recovery. More severe illness also results from other causes of weakened defenses, such as from severe stress, immunosuppressant medications, and severe intercurrent illnesses. **This is why steroids and other immunosuppressive medications are absolutely contraindicated in Lyme. This also includes intra-articular steroids.**

Many collateral conditions result in those who have been chronically ill so it is not surprising that damage to virtually all bodily systems can result. Therefore to fully recover not only do all of the active infections have to be treated, but all of these other issues must be addressed in a thorough and systematic manner. *No single treatment or medication will result in full recovery of the more ill patient. Only by addressing all of these issues and engineering treatments and solutions for all of them will we be able to restore full health to our patients.* Likewise, a patient will not recover unless they are completely compliant with every single aspect of the treatment plan. This must be emphasized to the patient, often on repeated occasions.

It is clear that in the great majority of patients, chronic Lyme is a disease affecting predominantly the nervous system. Thus, careful evaluation may include neuropsychiatric testing, SPECT and MRI brain scans, CSF analysis when appropriate, regular input from Lyme-aware neurologists and psychiatrists, pain clinics, and occasionally specialists in psychopharmacology.

HYPOTHALAMIC-PITUITARY AXIS

As an extension of the effect of chronic Lyme Disease on the central nervous system, there often is a deleterious effect on the hypothalamic-pituitary axis. Varying degrees of pituitary insufficiency are being seen in these patients, the correction of which has resulted in restoration of energy, stamina and libido, and resolution of persistent hypotension. Unfortunately, not all specialists recognize pituitary insufficiency, partly because of the difficulty in making the laboratory diagnosis. However, the potential benefits of diagnosing and treating this justify the effort needed for full evaluation. Interestingly, in a significant number of these patients, successful treatment of the infections can result in a reversal of the hormonal dysfunction, and hormone replacement therapies can be tapered off!

CO-INFECTION

A huge body of research and clinical experience has demonstrated the nearly universal phenomenon in chronic Lyme patients of co-infection with multiple tick-borne pathogens. These patients have been shown to potentially carry Babesia species, Bartonella-like organisms, Ehrlichia, Anaplasma, Mycoplasma, and viruses. Rarely, yeast forms have been detected in peripheral blood. At one point even nematodes were said to be a tick-borne pathogen. Studies have shown that co-infection results in a more severe clinical presentation, with more organ damage, and the pathogens become more difficult to eradicate. In addition, it is known that Babesia infections, like Lyme Borreliosis, are immunosuppressive.

There are changes in the clinical presentation of the co-infected patient as compared to when each infection is present individually. There may be different symptoms and atypical signs. There may be decreased reliability of standard diagnostic tests, and most importantly, there is recognition that chronic, persistent forms of each of these infections do indeed exist. As time goes by, I am convinced that even more pathogens will be found.

Therefore, real, clinical Lyme as we have come to know it, especially the later and more severe presentations, probably represents a mixed infection with many complicating factors. I will leave to the reader the implications of how this may explain the discrepancy between laboratory study of pure Borrelia infections, and what front line physicians have been seeing for years in real patients.

I must very strongly emphasize that all diagnoses of tick-borne infections remains a clinical one. Clinical clues will be presented later in this monograph, but testing information is briefly summarized below.

In **Lyme Borreliosis**, western blot is the preferred serologic test. Antigen detection tests (antigen capture and PCR), although insensitive, are very specific and are especially helpful in evaluating the seronegative patient and those still ill or relapsing after therapy. Often, these antigen detection tests are the only positive markers of Bb infection, as seronegativity has been reported to occur in as many as 30% to 50% of cases. Nevertheless, active LB can be present even if all of these tests are non-reactive! Clinical diagnosis is therefore required.

In **Babesiosis**, no single test is reliable enough to be used alone. Only in early infections (less than two weeks duration) can the standard blood smear be helpful. In later stages, one can use serology, PCR, and fluorescent in-situ hybridization ("FISH") assay. Unfortunately, many other protozoans can be found in ticks, most likely representing species other than *B. microti*, yet commercial tests for only B. microti and B duncani (Formerly known as WA-1) are available at this time! In other words, the patient may have an infection that cannot be tested for. Here, as in Borrelia, clinical assessment is the primary diagnostic tool.

In **Ehrlichiosis and Anaplasmosis**, by definition you must test for both the monocytic and granulocytic forms. This may be accomplished by blood smear, PCR and serology. Many presently uncharacterized Ehrlichia-like organisms can be found in ticks and may not be picked up by currently available assays, so in this illness too, these tests are only an adjunct in making the diagnosis. Rarely, Rocky Mountain Spotted Fever can coexist, and even be chronic. Fortunately, treatment regimens are similar for all agents in this group.

In **Bartonella**, use both serology and PCR. PCR can be performed not only on blood and CSF, but as in LB, can be performed on biopsy specimens. Unfortunately, in my experience, these tests, even when both types are done, will presently miss over half the cases diagnosed clinically.

Frequent exposures to **Mycoplasmas** are common, resulting in a high prevalence of seropositivity, so the best way to confirm active infection is by PCR.

Chronic viral infections may be active in the chronic patient, due to their weakened immune response. PCR testing, and not serologies, should be used for diagnosis. Commonly seen viruses include HHV-6, CMV, and EBV.

COLLATERAL CONDITIONS
Experience has shown that collateral conditions exist in those who have been ill a long time. The evaluation should include testing both for differential diagnosis and for uncovering other subtle abnormalities that may coexist.

Test **B12 levels**, and be prepared to aggressively treat with parenteral formulations. If neurologic involvement is severe, then consideration should be given to treatment with methylcobalamin (as outlined below in the section on nutritional support).

Magnesium deficiency is very often present and quite severe. Hyperreflexia, muscle twitches, myocardial irritability, poor stamina and recurrent tight muscle spasms are clues to this deficiency. Magnesium is predominantly an intracellular ion, so blood level testing is of little value. Oral preparations are acceptable for maintenance, but those with severe deficiencies need additional, parenteral dosing: 1 gram IV or IM at least once a week until neuromuscular irritability has cleared.

Pituitary and other endocrine abnormalities are far more common than generally realized. Evaluate fully, including growth hormone levels. Quite often, a full battery of provocative tests is in order to fully define the problem. When testing the thyroid, measure free T3 and free T4 levels and TSH, and nuclear scanning and testing for autoantibodies may be necessary.

Activation of the **inflammatory cascade** has been implicated in blockade of cellular hormone receptors. One example of this is insulin resistance; clinical hypothyroidism can result from receptor blockade and thus hypothyroidism can exist despite normal serum hormone levels. These may partly account for the dyslipidemia and weight gain that is noted in 80% of chronic Lyme patients. In addition to measuring free T3 and T4 levels, check basal A.M. body temperatures. If hypothyroidism is found, you may need to treat with both T3 and T4 preparations until blood levels of both are normalized. To ensure sustained levels, when T3 is prescribed, have it compounded in a time-release form.

Neurally mediated hypotension (NMH) is not uncommon. Symptoms can include palpitations, lightheadedness and shakiness especially after exertion and prolonged standing, heat intolerance, dizziness, fainting (or near fainting), *and an unavoidable need to sit or lie down*. It is often confused with hypoglycemia, which it mimics. NMH can result from autonomic neuropathy and endocrine dyscrasias. If NMH is present, treatment can dramatically lessen fatigue, palpitations and wooziness, and increase stamina. NMH is diagnosed by tilt table testing. This test should be done by a cardiologist and include Isuprel challenge. This will demonstrate not only if NMH is present, but also the relative contributions of hypovolemia and sympathetic dysfunction. Immediate supportive therapy is based on blood volume expansion (increased sodium and fluid intake and possibly Florinef plus potassium). If not sufficient, beta blockade may be added based on response to the Isuprel challenge. The long term solution involves restoring proper hormone levels and treating the Lyme to address this and the autonomic dysfunction.

SPECT scanning of the brain- Unlike MRI and CT scans, which show structure, SPECT scans show function. Therefore SPECT scans give us information unattainable through X-rays, CT scans, MRI's, or even spinal taps. In the majority of chronic Lyme Borreliosis patients, these scans are abnormal. Although not diagnostic of Lyme specifically, if the scan is abnormal, the scan can not only quantify the abnormalities, but the pattern can help to differentiate medical from psychiatric causes of these changes. Furthermore, repeat scans after a course of treatment can be used to assess treatment efficacy. Note that improvement in scans lag behind clinical improvement by many months.

If done by knowledgeable radiologists using high-resolution equipment, scanning will show characteristic abnormalities in Lyme encephalopathy- global hypoperfusion (may be homogenous or heterogeneous). What these scans demonstrate is neuronal dysfunction and/or varying degrees of cerebrolvascular insufficiency. If necessary, to assess the relative contributions of these two processes, the SPECT scan can be done before and after acetazolamide. If the post acetazolamide scan shows significant reversibility of the abnormalities, then vasoconstriction is present, and can be treated with vasodilators, which may clear some cognitive symptoms. Therapy can include acetazolamide, serotonin agonists and even Ginkgo biloba, provided it is of pharmaceutical quality. Therapeutic trials of these may be needed.

Acetazolamide should not be given if there is severe kidney/liver disease, electrolyte abnormalities, pregnancy, sulfa allergy, recent stroke, or if the patient is taking high dose aspirin treatment

LYME BORRELIOSIS

DIAGNOSTIC HINTS
Lyme Borreliosis (LB) is diagnosed clinically, as no currently available test, no matter the source or type, is definitive in ruling in or ruling out infection with these pathogens, or whether these infections are responsible

for the patient's symptoms. The entire clinical picture must be taken into account, including a search for concurrent conditions and alternate diagnoses, and other reasons for some of the presenting complaints. Often, much of the diagnostic process in late, disseminated Lyme involves ruling out other illnesses and defining the extent of damage that might require separate evaluation and treatment.

Consideration should be given to tick exposure, rashes (even atypical ones), evolution of typical symptoms in a previously asymptomatic individual, and results of tests for tick-borne pathogens. Another very important factor is response to treatment- presence or absence of Jarisch Herxheimer-like reactions, the classic four-week cycle of waxing and waning of symptoms, and improvement with therapy.

ERYTHEMA MIGRANS
Erythema migrans (EM) is diagnostic of Bb infection, but is present in *fewer than half*. Even if present, it may go unnoticed by the patient. It is an erythematous, centrifugally expanding lesion that is raised and may be warm. Rarely there is mild stinging or pruritus. The EM rash will begin four days to several weeks after the bite, and may be associated with constitutional symptoms. Multiple lesions are present less than 10% of the time, but do represent disseminated disease. Some lesions have an atypical appearance and skin biopsy specimens may be helpful. When an ulcerated or vesicular center is seen, this may represent a mixed infection, involving other organisms besides B. burgdorferi.

After a tick bite, serologic tests (ELISA. IFA, western blots, etc.) are not expected to become positive until several weeks have passed. Therefore, if EM is present, treatment must begin immediately, and one should not wait for results of Borrelia tests. You should not miss the chance to treat early disease, for this is when the success rate is the highest. Indeed, many knowledgeable clinicians will not even order a Borrelia test in this circumstance.

DIAGNOSING LATER DISEASE
When reactive, serologies indicate exposure only and do not directly indicate whether the spirochete is now currently present. Because Bb serologies often give inconsistent results, test at well-known reference laboratories. The suggestion that two-tiered testing, utilizing an ELISA as a screening tool, followed, if positive, by a confirmatory western blot, is illogical in this illness. The ELISA is not sensitive enough to serve as an adequate screen, and there are many patients with Lyme who test negative by ELISA yet have fully diagnostic western blots. I therefore recommend against using the ELISA. The newly available C6 ELISA appears to be no more sensitive than standard ELISAs, and in my experience there are even more false negative C6 assays in late disease than in earlier stages of the illness. I therefore do not recommend or use this type ELISA either. Instead, order IgM and IgG western blots- but be aware that in late disease there may be repeatedly peaking IgM's and therefore a reactive IgM may not differentiate early from late disease, but it does suggest an active infection. When late cases of LB are seronegative, 36% will transiently become seropositive at the completion of successful therapy. In chronic Lyme Borreliosis, the CD-57 count is both useful and important (see below).

Western blots are reported by showing which bands are reactive. 41KD bands appear the earliest but can cross react with other spirochetes. The 18KD, 23-25KD (Osp C), 31KD (Osp A), 34KD (Osp B), 37KD, 39KD, 83KD and the 93KD bands are the species-specific ones, but appear later or may not appear at all. You should see at least the 41KD and one of the specific bands. 55KD, 60KD, 66KD, and 73KD are nonspecific and nondiagnostic.

PCR tests are now available, and although they are very specific, sensitivity remains poor, possibly less than 30%. This is because Bb causes a deep tissue infection and is only transiently found in body humors. Therefore, just as in routine blood culturing, multiple specimens must be collected to increase yield; a negative result does not rule out infection, but a positive one is significant. You can test whole blood, buffy coat, serum, urine, spinal and other body fluids, and tissue biopsies. Several blood PCRs can be done, or you can run PCRs on whole blood, serum and urine simultaneously at a time of active symptoms. The patient should be antibiotic-free for at least six weeks before testing to obtain the highest yield.

Antigen capture is becoming more widely available, and can be done on urine, CSF, and synovial fluid. Sensitivity is still low (on the order of 30%), but specificity is high (greater than 90%).

Spinal taps are not routinely recommended, as a negative tap does not rule out Lyme. Antibodies to Bb are mostly found in Lyme meningitis, and are rarely seen in non-meningitic CNS infection, including advanced encephalopathy. Even in meningitis, antibodies are detected in the CSF in less than 13% of patients with late disease! Therefore, spinal taps are only performed on patients with pronounced neurological manifestations in whom the diagnosis is uncertain, if they are seronegative, or are still significantly symptomatic after completion of treatment. When done, the goal is to rule out other conditions, and to determine if Bb (and Bartonella) antigens or nucleic acids are present. It is especially important to look for elevated protein and white cells, which would dictate the need for more aggressive therapy, as well as the opening pressure, which can be elevated and add to headaches, especially in children.

I strongly urge you to **biopsy** all unexplained skin lesions/rashes and perform PCR and careful histology. You will need to alert the pathologist to look for spirochetes.

THE CD-57 TEST
Our ability to measure CD-57 counts represents a breakthrough in LB diagnosis and treatment.

Chronic LB infections are known to suppress the immune system and can decrease the quantity of the CD-57 subset of the natural killer cells. As in HIV infection, where abnormally low T-cell counts are routinely used as a marker of how active that infection is, in LB we can use the degree of decrease of the CD-57 count to indicate how active the Lyme infection is and whether, after treatment ends, a relapse is likely to occur. It can even be used as a simple, inexpensive screening test, because at this point we believe that only Borrelia will depress the CD-57. Thus, a sick patient with a high CD-57 is probably ill with something other than Lyme, such as a co-infection.

When this test is run by LabCorp (the currently preferred lab, as published studies were based on their assays), we want our Lyme patients to measure above 60; a normal count is above 200. There generally is some degree of fluctuation of this count over time, and the number does not progressively increase as treatment proceeds. Instead, it remains low until the LB infection is controlled, and then it will jump. If the CD-57 count is not in the normal range when a course of antibiotics is ended, then a relapse will almost certainly occur.

CHECK LIST OF **CURRENT** SYMPTOMS: This is not meant to be used as a diagnostic scheme, but is provided to streamline the office interview. Note the format- complaints referable to specific organ systems and specific co-infections are clustered to clarify diagnoses and to better display multisystem involvement.

Have you had any of the following in relation to this illness? (CIRCLE "NO" OR "YES")

Tick bite	N Y	*"EM" rash (discrete circle)*	N Y
Spotted rash over large area	N Y	*Linear, red streaks*	N Y

SYMPTOM OR SIGN	CURRENT SEVERITY				CURRENT FREQUENCY				
	NONE	MILD	MODERATE	SEVERE	NA	NEVER	OCCASIONAL	OFTEN	CONSTANT
Persistent swollen glands									
Sore throat									
Fevers									
Sore soles, esp. in the AM									
Joint pain									
Fingers, toes									
Ankles, wrists									
Knees, elbows									
Hips, shoulders									
Joint swelling									
Fingers, toes									
Ankles, wrists									
Knees, elbows									
Hips, shoulders									
Unexplained back pain									
Stiffness of the joints or back									
Muscle pain or cramps									
Obvious muscle weakness									
Twitching of the face or other muscles									
Confusion, difficulty thinking									
Difficulty with concentration, reading, problem absorbing new information									
Word search, name block									
Forgetfulness, poor short term memory, poor attention									
Disorientation: getting lost, going to wrong places									
Speech errors- wrong word, misspeaking									
Mood swings, irritability, depression									
Anxiety, panic attacks									
Psychosis (hallucinations, delusions, paranoia, bipolar)									
Tremor									
Seizures									
Headache									
Light sensitivity									
Sound sensitivity									
Vision: double, blurry, floaters									
Ear pain									

SYMPTOM OR SIGN	CURRENT SEVERITY				CURRENT FREQUENCY				
	NONE	MILD	MODERATE	SEVERE	NA	NEVER	OCCASIONAL	OFTEN	CONSTANT
Hearing: buzzing, ringing, decreased hearing									
Increased motion sickness, vertigo, spinning									
Off balance, "tippy" feeling									
Lightheadedness, wooziness, unavoidable need to sit or lie									
Tingling, numbness, burning or stabbing sensations, shooting pains, skin hypersensitivity									
Facial paralysis-Bell's Palsy									
Dental pain									
Neck creaks and cracks, stiffness, neck pain									
Fatigue, tired, poor stamina									
Insomnia, fractionated sleep, early awakening									
Excessive night time sleep									
Napping during the day									
Unexplained weight gain									
Unexplained weight loss									
Unexplained hair loss									
Pain in genital area									
Unexplained menstrual irregularity									
Unexplained milk production; breast pain									
Irritable bladder or bladder dysfunction									
Erectile dysfunction									
Loss of libido									
Queasy stomach or nausea									
Heartburn, stomach pain									
Constipation									
Diarrhea									
Low abdominal pain, cramps									
Heart murmur or valve prolapse?									
Heart palpitations or skips									
"Heart block" on EKG									
Chest wall pain or ribs sore									
Head congestion									
Breathlessness, "air hunger", unexplained chronic cough									
Night sweats									
Exaggerated symptoms or worse hangover from alcohol									
Symptom flares every 4 wks.									
Degree of disability									

DIAGNOSTIC CHECKLIST

To aid the clinician, a workable set of diagnostic criteria were developed with the input of dozens of front line physicians. The resultant document, refined over the years, has proven to be extremely useful not only to the clinician, but it also can help clarify the diagnosis for third party payers and utilization review committees. **It is important to note that the CDC's published reporting criteria are for surveillance only, not for diagnosis. They should not be misused in an effort to diagnose Lyme or set guidelines for insurance company acceptance of the diagnosis, nor be used to determine eligibility for coverage.**

LYME BORRELIOSIS DIAGNOSTIC CRITERIA   RELATIVE VALUE

Tick exposure in an endemic region....... 1
Historical facts and evolution of symptoms over time consistent with Lyme 2
Systemic signs & symptoms consistent with Bb infection (other potential diagnoses excluded):
      Single system, e.g., monoarthritis 1
      Two or more systems, e.g., monoarthritis and facial palsy.. 2
Erythema migrans, physician confirmed. 7
Acrodermatitis Chronica Atrophicans, biopsy confirmed 7
Seropositivity 3
Seroconversion on paired sera.. 4
Tissue microscopy, silver stain.. 3
Tissue microscopy, monoclonal immunofluorescence 4
Culture positivity 4
B. burgdorferi antigen recovery 4
B. burgdorferi DNA/RNA recovery 4

DIAGNOSIS

Lyme Borreliosis Highly Likely................ ....7 or above
Lyme Borreliosis Possible...... 5-6
Lyme Borreliosis Unlikely....... ... .4 or below

I suggest that when using these criteria, you state Lyme Borreliosis is "unlikely", "possible", or "highly likely" based upon the following criteria"- then list the criteria.

LYME DISEASE TREATMENT GUIDELINES

LYME BORRELIOSIS:

GENERAL INFORMATION
After a tick bite, Bb undergoes rapid hematogenous dissemination, and for example, can be found within the central nervous system as soon as *twelve hours* after entering the bloodstream. This is why even early infections require full dose antibiotic therapy with an agent able to penetrate all tissues in concentrations known to be bactericidal to the organism.

It has been shown that the longer a patient had been ill with LB prior to first definitive therapy, the longer the duration of treatment must be, and the need for more aggressive treatment increases.

More evidence has accumulated indicating the severe detrimental effects of the concurrent use of immunosuppressants including steroids in the patient with active B. burgdorferi infection. **Never give steroids or any other immunosuppressant to any patient who may even remotely be suffering from Lyme, or serious, permanent damage may result, especially if given for anything greater than a short course.** If immunosuppressive therapy is absolutely necessary, then potent antibiotic treatment should begin at least 48 hours prior to the immunosuppressants.

TREATMENT RESISTANCE
Bb contains beta lactamases and cephalosporinases, which, with some strains, may confer resistance to cephalosporins and penicillins. This is apparently a slowly acting enzyme system, and may be overcome by higher or more continuous drug levels especially when maintained by continuous infusions (cefotaxime) and by depot preparations (benzathine penicillin). Nevertheless, some penicillin and cephalosporin treatment failures do occur and have responded to sulbactam/ampicillin, imipenem, and vancomycin, which act through different cell wall mechanisms than the penicillins and the cephalosporins.

Vegetative endocarditis has been associated with Borrelia burgdorferi, but the vegetations may be too small to detect with echocardiography. Keep this in mind when evaluating patients with murmurs, as this may explain why some patients seem to continually relapse after even long courses of antibiotics.

COMBINATION THERAPY
Treatment of chronic Lyme usually requires combinations of antibiotics. There are four reasons for this:
1. TWO COMPARTMENTS- Bb can be found in both the fluid and the tissue compartments, yet no single antibiotic currently used to treat Bb infections will be effective in both compartments. This is one reason for the need to use combination therapy in the more ill patient. A logical combination might use, for example, azithromycin plus a penicillin.
2. INTRACELLULAR NICHE- Another reason, discussed below, is the fact that Bb can penetrate and remain viable within cells and evade the effects of extracellular agents. Typical combinations include an extracellular antibiotic, plus an intracellular agent such as an erythromycin derivative or metronidazole. Note that some experts discourage the co-administration of bactericidal plus bacteriostatic agents, thus the recommendation to avoid a cell wall drug combined with a tetracycline.
3. L-FORMS (SPHEROPLAST)- It has been recognized that B. burgdorferi can exist in at least two, and possibly three different morphologic forms: spirochete, spheroplast (or l-form), and the recently discovered cystic form (presently, there is controversy whether the cyst is different from the l-form). L-forms and cystic forms do not contain cell walls, and thus beta lactam antibiotics will not affect them. Spheroplasts seem to be susceptible to tetracyclines and the advanced erythromycin derivatives. Apparently, Bb can shift among the three forms during the course of the infection. Because of this, it may be necessary to cycle different classes of antibiotics and/or prescribe a combination of dissimilar agents.
4. CYSTIC FORM- When present in a hostile environment, such as growth medium lacking some nutrients, spinal fluid, or serum with certain antibiotics added, Bb can change from the spiral

form ("spirochete") into a cyst form. This cyst seems to be able to remain dormant, but when placed into an environment more favorable to its growth, Bb can revert into the spirochete form. The antibiotics commonly used for Lyme do not kill the cystic form of Bb. However, there is laboratory evidence that metronidazole and tinidazole will disrupt it. Therefore, the chronically infected patient who has resistant disease may need to have metronidazole (or tinidazole) added to the regimen. More details are provided in the section on treatment options.

BORRELIA NEUROTOXIN (With thanks to Dr. Shoemaker)

Two groups have reported evidence that Borrelia, like several other bacteria, produce neurotoxins. These compounds reportedly can cause many of the symptoms of encephalopathy, cause an ongoing inflammatory reaction manifested as some of the virus-like symptoms common in late Lyme, and also potentially interfere with hormone action by blocking hormone receptors. At this time, there is no assay available to detect whether this compound is present, nor can the amount of toxin be quantified. Indirect measures are currently employed, such as measures of cytokine activation and hormone resistance. A visual contrast sensitivity test (VCS test) reportedly is quite useful in documenting CNS effects of the neurotoxin, and to follow effects of treatment. This test is available at some centers and on the internet.

It has been said that the longer one is ill with Lyme, the more neurotoxin is present in the body. It probably is stored in fatty tissues, and once present, persists for a very long time. This may be because of enterohepatic circulation, where the toxin is excreted via the bile into the intestinal tract, but then is reabsorbed from the intestinal tract back into the blood stream. This forms the basis for treatment.

Two prescription medications that can bind these toxins include cholestyramine resin and Welchol pills. When take orally in generous amounts, the neurotoxin present in the intestinal tract binds to the resin, is trapped, and then excreted. Thus, over several weeks, the level of neurotoxin is depleted and clinical improvement can be seen. Current experience is that improvement is first seen in three weeks, and treatment can continue for a month or more. Retreatment is always possible.

These medications may bind not only toxins but also many drugs and vitamin supplements. Therefore no other oral medications or supplements should be taken from a half hour before, to two hours after a dose of one of these fiber agents.

Cholestyramine should be taken two to four times daily, and Welchol is prescribed at three pills twice daily. While the latter is obviously much simpler to use, it is less effective than cholestyramine. The main side effects are bloating and constipation, best handled with increased fluid intake and gentle laxatives.

TREATING LYME BORRELIOSIS

LYME DISEASE TREATMENT INFORMATION

There is no universally effective antibiotic for treating LB. The choice of medication used and the dosage prescribed will vary for different people based on multiple factors. These include duration and severity of illness, presence of co-infections, immune deficiencies, prior significant immunosuppressant use while infected, age, weight, gastrointestinal function, blood levels achieved, and patient tolerance. Doses found to be effective clinically are often higher than those recommended in older texts. This is due to deep tissue penetration by Bb, its presence in the CNS including the eye, within cells, within tendons, and because very few of the many strains of this organism now known to exist have been studied for antibiotic susceptibility. In addition, all animal studies of susceptibility to date have only addressed early disease in models that behave differently than human hosts. Therefore, begin with a regimen appropriate to the setting, and if necessary, modify it over time based upon antibiotic blood level measurements and clinical response.

ANTIBIOTICS

There are four types of antibiotics in general use for Bb treatment. The TETRACYCLINES (tetracycline, minocycline and doxycycline, but not tigecycline- see below), are bacteriostatic unless given in high doses. If high blood levels are not attained, treatment failures in early and late disease are common. However, these high doses can be difficult to tolerate. For example, doxycycline can be very effective but only if adequate blood levels are achieved either by high oral doses (300 to 600 mg daily) or by parenteral administration. Kill kinetics indicate that a large spike in blood and tissue levels is more effective than sustained levels, which is why with doxycycline, oral doses of 200 mg bid is more effective than 100 mg qid. Likewise, this is why IV doses of 400 mg once a day is more effective than any oral regimen. However, the newly available, parenteral-only tetracycline, tigecycline, represents a true advance, in that it inhibits efflux of the antibiotic (basically a minocycline derivative) out of the host cells, thus achieving far better results than even parenteral doxycycline. As with all tetracyclines, nausea remains the primary and use-limiting side effect of this drug.

PENICILLINS are bactericidal. As would be expected in managing an infection with a gram negative organism such as Bb, amoxicillin has been shown to be more effective than oral penicillin V. With cell wall agents such as the penicillins, kill kinetics indicate that sustained bactericidal levels are needed for 72 hours to be effective. Thus the goal is to try to achieve sustained blood and tissue levels. However, since blood levels are extremely variable among patients, peak and trough levels should be measured (for details, refer to the antibiotic dosage table). Because of its short half-life and need for high levels, amoxicillin is usually administered along with probenecid. An extended release formulation of amoxicillin+clavulanate ("Augmentin XR") may also be considered if adequate trough levels are difficult to attain. An attractive alternative is benzathine penicillin ("Bicillin-LA"- see below). This is an intramuscular depot injection, and although doses are relatively small, the sustained blood and tissue levels are what make this preparation so effective.

CEPHALOSPORINS must be of advanced generation: first generation drugs are rarely effective and second generation drugs are comparable to amoxicillin and doxycycline both in-vitro and in-vivo. Third generation agents are currently the most effective of the cephalosporins because of their very low MBC's (0.06 for ceftriaxone), and relatively long half-life. Cephalosporins have been shown to be effective in penicillin and tetracycline failures. Cefuroxime axetil (Ceftin), a second generation agent, is also effective against staph and thus is useful in treating atypical erythema migrans that may represent a mixed infection that contains some of the more common skin pathogens in addition to Bb. Because this agent's G.I. side effects and high cost, it is not often used as first line drug. As with the penicillins, try to achieve high, sustained blood and tissue levels by frequent dosing and/or the use of probenecid. Measure peak and trough blood levels when possible.

When choosing a third generation cephalosporin, there are several points to remember: Ceftriaxone is administered twice daily (an advantage for home therapy), but has 95% biliary excretion and can crystallize in the biliary tree with resultant colic and possible cholecystitis. GI excretion results in a large impact on gut flora. Biliary and superinfection problems with ceftriaxone can be lessened if this drug is given in interrupted courses (known commonly as "pulse therapy"- refer to chapter on this on page 20), so the current recommendation is to administer it four days in a row each week. Cefotaxime, which must be given at least every eight hours or as a continuous infusion, is less convenient, but as it has only 5% biliary excretion, it never causes biliary concretions, and may have less impact on gut flora.

ERYTHROMYCIN has been shown to be almost ineffective as monotherapy. The azalide azithromycin is somewhat more effective but only minimally so when given orally. As an IV drug, much better results are seen. Clarithromycin is more effective as an oral agent than azithromycin, but can be difficult to tolerate due to its tendency to promote yeast overgrowth, bad aftertaste, and poor GI tolerance at the high doses needed. These problems are much less severe with the ketolide telithromycin, which is generally well tolerated.

Erythromycins (and the advanced generation derivatives mentioned above) have impressively low MBCs and they do concentrate in tissues and penetrate cells, so they theoretically should be ideal agents. So why is it that erythromycin is ineffective, and why have initial clinical results with azithromycin (and to a lesser degree, clarithromycin) been disappointing? It has been suggested that when Bb is within a cell, it is held within a vacuole and bathed in fluid of low pH, and this acidity may inactivate azithromycin and clarithromycin. Therefore, they are administered concurrently with hydroxychloroquine or amantadine, which raise vacuolar pH, rendering these antibiotics more effective. It is not known whether this same technique will make erythromycin a more effective antibiotic in LB. Another alternative is to administer azithromycin parenterally. Results are excellent, but expect to see abrupt Jarisch-Herxheimer reactions.

Telithromycin, on the other hand, is stable in the intracellular acid environment, which may be why this is currently by far the most effective drug of this class, and may replace the others in the majority of patients with LB. Likewise, there is no need to co-administer amantadine or hydroxychloroquine. This antibiotic has other advantages- it has been engineered to prevent drug resistance, has almost no negative impact on E. coli in the intestinal tract (hopefully minimizing the risk for diarrhea), and it can be taken with or without food.

However, there are disadvantages:
1. May interact with a wide variety of medications because it is an inhibitor of the cytochrome CYP3A4. It is vital that this be taken into account as many Lyme patients take a variety of medications concurrently, and often from several practitioners.
2. May lengthen the QT interval. This should be measured prior to prescribing this drug, and if borderline, rechecked after it is begun.
3. Can transiently cause blurry vision, delayed accommodation, and even double vision.
4. Liver enzymes may become elevated. Blood tests should be done regularly to monitor this.
5. The usual precautions of any antibiotic also still apply- risk for allergy, stomach upset, Herxheimer reactions, etc.

QTc INTERVAL
- QTc is the QT corrected for heart rate
- Measure the precordial lead that has the best T wave (usually V-2 or V-5)
- Measure from the start of the Q wave to the end of the T wave
- QT interval is inversely related to the heart rate (slow pulse results in a longer QT)
- $QTc = QT \div \sqrt{RR}$ interval
- Normals: Females <450 ms, Males < 470 ms
- Want K+ > 4.0, Mg++ > 2.0; avoid hypocalcemia

METRONIDAZOLE (Flagyl) When present in a hostile environment, such as growth medium lacking some nutrients, spinal fluid, or serum with certain antibiotics added, Bb can change into a cyst form. This cyst seems to be able to remain dormant, but when placed into an environment more favorable to its growth, the cyst can revert into the spirochete form. The conventional antibiotics used for Lyme, such as the penicillins, cephalosporins, etc do not kill the cystic form of Bb, yet there is laboratory evidence that metronidazole will kill it. Therefore, the trend now is to treat the chronically infected patient who has resistant disease by combining metronidazole with one or two other antibiotics to target all forms of Bb. Because there is laboratory evidence that tetracyclines may inhibit the effect of Flagyl, this class of medication should not be used in these two- and three-drug regimens. Some clinicians favor tinidazole as this may be equally effective but result in fewer side effects. However, this has yet to be documented.

Important precautions:
1. Pregnancy while on Flagyl is not advised, as there is a risk of birth defects.
2. No alcohol consumption! A severe, "Antabuse" reaction will occur, consisting of severe nausea, flushing, headache, and other symptoms.
3. Yeast overgrowth is especially common. A strict anti-yeast regimen must be followed.
4. Flagyl can be irritative to the nervous system- in the short term, it may cause irritability, "spacey" feelings, etc. Longer term, it can affect the peripheral nerves, causing tingles, numbness, etc. If mild, a change in dose may be required. Often, extra vitamin B can clear these symptoms. If the nerve symptoms persist or are strong, then metronidazole must be discontinued or these symptoms may become very long lasting.
5. Strong Herxheimer-like reactions are seen in almost everyone.

RIFAMPIN is a well-known antibiotic that has been in use for many decades. It is primarily used to treat tuberculosis, but also has been used in other conditions, such as prevention of meningitis in those exposed, for treating resistant Staph, etc. Potentially, rifampin may be effective in treating Bartonella, Ehrlichia, Mycoplasma, and Borrelia. There are as yet no formal clinical studies on the use of this medication in these illnesses, but many patients have been treated with rifampin and have had favorable results. When used, regular blood tests (CBC, liver enzymes) are usually performed to monitor for side effects. Rifampin can also discolor urine, tears and sweat (brownish-orange). It may also stain some types of water-permeable contact lenses. Taking rifampin during pregnancy is not advised. Finally, because this drug is an inducer of cytochromes (CYP3A4), co-administration with other medications may result in lower and more brief blood levels of the co-administered drug. Thus, be aware of these potential drug interactions.

BENZATHINE PENICILLIN Comparative studies published by Fallon et. al. at Columbia University have shown that parenteral therapy is superior to oral therapy in chronic patients. Options include intramuscular long acting penicillin G (benzathine penicillin, or "Bicillin-LA") or intravenous antibiotics.

For an antibiotic in the penicillin class to be effective, time-killing curves show that significant levels of antibiotic must be sustained for 72 hours. Bicillin LA is a sustained release formulation that meets these criteria.

Published studies in children and adults, combined with over a decade of experience with this therapy by front line, Lyme-treating physicians have established the efficacy, safety and usefulness of this medication. In many patients it is more effective than oral antibiotics for treating Lyme, and compares closely to intravenous therapy in terms of efficacy if the dose is high enough.

It is usually administered three or four times weekly for six to twelve months. It has the advantage of being relatively inexpensive, free of gastrointestinal side effects, unlikely to promote the overgrowth of yeast, and has an excellent safety record spanning many decades.

Finally, an added plus is that family members can be trained to administer this treatment at home.

CEFTRIAXONE TREATMENT A subset of patients who have severe, longstanding illness due to Borrelia burgdorferi carry persistent infection despite having previously received antibiotic treatments which have eliminated the disease in less ill individuals. The mechanism for such persistence has been the subject of many peer reviewed articles. They include persistence of B. burgdorferi in protective niches, inhibition and lysis of lymphocytes, survival in phagocytic vacuoles, antigenic shifts, slow growth, shifting into alternate forms, and dormancy and latency.

One successful approach in the more ill patient, published in the early 1990s, is to use higher doses of ceftriaxone in a pulsed-dose regimen. Since then, clinical experience has expanded upon this concept, and at the MLDA Lyme Congress in September, 2002, Cichon presented data on a pulsed, high dose regimen which supports and refines this concept. This regimen is now considered the current standard of care in the use of ceftriaxone.

Treatment with ceftriaxone is dosed at 4 grams daily- given either as 2 grams IV twice daily, or 4 grams slowly once a day, four days in a row each week, usually for 14 or more weeks. Such a regimen is not only more effective in the Chronic Lyme patient, but regular interruptions in treatment lessen the potential complications of intensive antibiotic therapy with ceftriaxone, such as biliary sludging and colitis. Hence a more effective, safer regimen that by virtue of the treatment breaks, is less costly and affords the patient a more acceptable lifestyle. IV access with a heparin lock becomes possible (and preferred).

COURSE DURING THERAPY
As the spirochete has a very long generation time (12 to 24 hours *in vitro* and possibly much longer in living systems) and may have periods of dormancy, during which time antibiotics will not kill the organism, treatment has to be continued for a long period of time to eradicate all the active symptoms and prevent a relapse, especially in late infections. If treatment is discontinued before all symptoms of active infection have cleared, the patient will remain ill and possibly relapse further. In general, early LB is treated for four to six weeks, and late LB usually requires a minimum of four to six months of continuous treatment. All patients respond differently and therapy must be individualized. It is not uncommon for a patient who has been ill for many years to require open ended treatment regimens; indeed, some patients will require ongoing maintenance therapy for years to remain well.

Several days after the onset of appropriate antibiotic therapy, symptoms often flare due to lysis of the spirochetes with release of increased amount of antigenic material and possibly bacterial toxins. This is referred to as a Jarisch Herxheimer-like reaction. Because it takes 48 to 72 hours of therapy to initiate bacterial killing, the Herxheimer reaction is therefore delayed. This is unlike syphilis, in which these reactions can occur within hours.

It has been observed that symptoms will flare in cycles every four weeks. It is thought that this reflects the organism's cell cycle, with the growth phase occurring once per month (intermittent growth is common in Borrelia species). As antibiotics will only kill bacteria during their growth phase, therapy is designed to bracket at least one whole generation cycle. This is why the minimum treatment duration should be at least four weeks. If the antibiotics are working, over time these flares will lessen in severity and duration. The very occurrence of ongoing monthly cycles indicates that living organisms are still present and that antibiotics should be continued.

With treatment, these monthly symptom flares are exaggerated and presumably represent recurrent Herxheimer-like reactions as Bb enters its vulnerable growth phase and then are lysed. For unknown reasons, the worst occurs at the fourth week of treatment. Observation suggest that the more severe this reaction, the higher the germ load, and the more ill the patient. In those with long-standing highly symptomatic disease who are on I.V. therapy, the week-four flare can be very severe, similar to a serum sickness reaction, and be associated with transient leucopenia and/or elevations in liver enzymes. If this happens, decrease the dose temporarily, or interrupt treatment for several days, then resume with a lower dose. If you are able to continue or resume therapy, then patients continue to improve. Those whose treatment is stopped and not restarted at this point usually will need retreatment in the future due to ongoing or recurrent symptoms because the infection was not eradicated. Patients on I.V. therapy who have a strong reaction at the fourth week will need to continue parenteral antibiotics for several months, for when this monthly reaction finally lessens in severity, then oral or IM medications can be substituted. Indeed, it is just this observation that guides the clinician in determining the endpoint of I.V. treatment. In general, I.V. therapy is given until there is a clear positive response, and then treatment is changed to IM or po until free of signs of active infection for 4 to 8 weeks. Some patients, however, will not respond to IM or po treatment and I.V. therapy will have to be used throughout. As mentioned earlier, leucopenia may be a sign of persistent Ehrlichiosis, so be sure to look into this.

Repeated treatment failures should alert the clinician to the possibility of an otherwise inapparent immune deficiency, and a workup for this may be advised. Obviously, evaluation for co-infection should be performed, and a search for other or concurrent diagnoses needs to be entertained.

There are three things that will predict treatment failure regardless of which regimen is chosen: Non-compliance, alcohol use, and sleep deprivation. Advise them to take a break when (or ideally before) the inevitable mid afternoon fatigue sets in (napping is encouraged).

All patients must keep a carefully detailed daily diary of their symptoms to help us document the presence of the classic four week cycle, judge the effects of treatment, and determine treatment endpoint. One must follow such diaries, temperature readings in late afternoon, physical findings, notes from physical therapists, and cognitive testing to best judge when to change or end antibiotics.

Remember- there currently is no test for cure, so this clinical follow-up assumes a major role in Lyme Disease care.

ANTIBIOTIC CHOICES AND DOSES

ORAL THERAPY: Always check blood levels when using agents marked with an *, and adjust dose to achieve a peak level above ten and a trough greater than three. Because of this, the doses listed below may have to be raised. Consider Doxycycline first in early Lyme due to concern for Ehrlichia co-infections.

*Amoxicillin- Adults: 1g q8h plus probenecid 500mg q8h; doses up to 6 grams daily are
often needed

Pregnancy: 1g q6h and adjust.

Children: 50 mg/kg/day divided into q8h doses.

*Doxycycline- Adults: 200 mg bid with food; doses of up to 600 mg daily are often needed, as doxycycline is only effective at high blood levels. Not for children or in pregnancy.

If levels are too low at tolerated doses, give parenterally or change to another drug.

*Cefuroxime axetil- Oral alternative that may be effective in amoxicillin and doxycycline failures. Useful in EM rashes co-infected with common skin pathogens.

Adults and pregnancy: 1g q12h and adjust. Children: 125 to 500 mg q12h based on weight.

Tetracycline- Adults only, and not in pregnancy. 500 mg tid to qid

Erythromycin- Poor response and not recommended.

Azithromycin- Adults: 500 to 1200 mg/d. Adolescents: 250 to 500 mg/d

Add hydroxychloroquine, 200-400 mg/d, or amantadine 100-200 mg/d

Cannot be used in pregnancy or in younger children.

Overall, poor results when administered orally

Clarithromycin- Adults: 250 to 500 mg q6h plus hydroxychloroquine, 200-400 mg/d, or amantadine 100-200 mg/d. Cannot be used in pregnancy or in younger children.

Clinically more effective than azithromycin

Telithromycin- Adolescents and adults: 800 mg once daily

Do not need to use amantadine or hydroxychloroquine

So far, the most effective drug of this class, and possibly the best oral agent if tolerated. Expect strong and quite prolonged Herxheimer reactions.

Must watch for drug interactions (CYP3A-4 inhibitor), check the QTc interval, and monitor liver enzymes.

Not to be used in pregnancy.

*Augmentin- Standard Augmentin cannot exceed three tablets daily due to the clavulanate, thus is given with amoxicillin, so that the total dose of the amoxicillin component is as listed above for amoxicillin. This combination can be effective when Bb beta lactamase is felt to be significant.

*Augmentin XR 1000- This is a time-release formulation and thus is a better choice than standard Augmentin.

Dose- 1000 mg q 8 h, to 2000 mg q 12 h based on blood levels.

Chloramphenicol- Not recommended as not proven and potentially toxic.

Metronidazole: 500 to 1500 mg daily in divided doses. Non-pregnant adults only.

PARENTERAL THERAPY

Ceftriaxone- Risk of biliary sludging (therefore often Actigall is co-administered- one to three tablets daily).

Adults and pregnancy: 2g q12 h, 4 days in a row each week

Children: 75 mg/kg/day up to 2g/day

Cefotaxime- Comparable efficacy to ceftriaxone; no biliary complications.

Adults and pregnancy: 6g to 12g daily. Can be given q 8 h as divided doses, but a continuous infusion may be more efficacious. When exceeding 6 g daily, use pulsed-dose schedule

Children: 90 to 180 mg/kg/day dosed q6h (preferred) or q8h, not to exceed 12 g daily.

*Doxycycline- Requires central line as is caustic.

Surprisingly effective, probably because blood levels are higher when given parenterally and single large daily doses optimize kinetics of killing with this drug. Always measure blood levels.

Adults: Start at 400 mg q24h and adjust based on levels.

Cannot be used in pregnancy or in younger children.

Tigecycline- requires central line as is caustic

By far the most effective tetracycline, and very useful to also treat difficult intracellular co-infections

Cannot be used in pregnancy and in younger children

Dose is 50 mg IV q 12h.

Azithromycin- Requires central line as is caustic.

Dose: 500 to 1000 mg daily in adolescents and adults.

Penicillin G- IV penicillin G is minimally effective and not recommended.

Benzathine penicillin- Surprisingly effective IM alternative to oral therapy. May need to begin at lower doses as strong, prolonged (6 or more week) Herxheimer-like reactions have been observed.

Adults: 1.2 million U- three to four doses weekly.

Adolescents: 1.2 to 3.6 million U weekly.

May be used in pregnancy.

Vancomycin- observed to be one of the best drugs in treating Lyme, but potential toxicity limits its use. It is a perfect candidate for pulse therapy to minimize these concerns. Use standard doses and confirm levels.

Primaxin and Unisyn- similar in efficacy to cefotaxime, but often work when cephalosporins have failed.

Must be given q6 to q8 hours.

Cefuroxime- useful but not demonstrably better than ceftriaxone or cefotaxime.

*Ampicillin IV- more effective than penicillin G. Must be given q6 hours.

TREATMENT CATEGORIES

PROPHYLAXIS of high risk groups- education and preventive measures. Antibiotics are not given.

TICK BITES - Embedded Deer Tick With No Signs or Symptoms of Lyme (see appendix):

Decide to treat based on the type of tick, whether it came from an endemic area, how it was removed, and length of attachment (anecdotally, as little as four hours of attachment can transmit pathogens). The risk of transmission is greater if the tick is engorged, or of it was removed improperly allowing the tick's contents to spill into the bite wound. High-risk bites are treated as follows (remember the possibility of co-infection!):

1) Adults: Oral therapy for 28 days.

2) Pregnancy: Amoxicillin 1000 mg q6h for 6 weeks. Test for Babesia, Bartonella and Ehrlichia.

Alternative: Cefuroxime axetil 1000 mg q12h for 6 weeks.

3) Young Children: Oral therapy for 28 days.

EARLY LOCALIZED - Single erythema migrans with no constitutional symptoms:

1) Adults: oral therapy- must continue until symptom and sign free for at least one month, with a 6 week minimum.

2) Pregnancy: 1st and 2nd trimesters: I.V. X 30 days then oral X 6 weeks

3rd trimester: Oral therapy X 6+ weeks as above.

Any trimester- test for Babesia and Ehrlichia

3) Children: oral therapy for 6+ weeks.

DISSEMINATED DISEASE - Multiple lesions, constitutional symptoms, lymphadenopathy, or any other manifestations of dissemination.

EARLY DISSEMINATED: Milder symptoms present for less than one year and not complicated by immune deficiency or prior steroid treatment:

1) Adults: oral therapy until no active disease for 4 to 8 weeks (4-6 months typical)

2) Pregnancy: As in localized disease, but treat throughout pregnancy.

3) Children: Oral therapy with duration based upon clinical response.

PARENTERAL ALTERNATIVES for more ill patients and those unresponsive to or intolerant of oral medications:

1) Adults and children: I.V. therapy until clearly improved, with a 6 week minimum. Follow with oral

therapy or IM benzathine penicillin until no active disease for 6-8 weeks. I.V. may have to be resumed if oral or IM therapy fails.

2) Pregnancy: IV then oral therapy as above.

LATE DISSEMINATED: present greater than one year, more severely ill patients, and those with prior significant steroid therapy or any other cause of impaired immunity:

1) Adults and pregnancy: extended I.V. therapy (14 or more weeks), then oral or IM, if effective, to same endpoint. Combination therapy with at least two dissimilar antibiotics almost always needed.

2) Children: IV therapy for 6 or more weeks, then oral or IM follow up as above. Combination therapy usually needed.

CHRONIC LYME DISEASE (PERSISTENT/RECURRENT INFECTION)

By definition, this category consists of patients with active infection, of a more prolonged duration, who are more likely have higher spirochete loads, weaker defense mechanisms, possibly more virulent or resistant strains, and probably are significantly co-infected. Neurotoxins may also be significant in these patients. Search for and treat for all of these, and search for concurrent infections including viruses, chlamydias, and mycoplasmas. Be sure to do an endocrine workup if indicated. These patients require a full evaluation for all of these problems, and each abnormality must be addressed.

This group will most likely need parenteral therapy, especially high dose, pulsed therapy, and antibiotic combinations, including metronidazole. Antibiotic therapy will need to continue for many months, and the antibiotics may have to be changed periodically to break plateaus in recovery. Be vigilant for treatment-related problems such as antibiotic-associated colitis, yeast overgrowth, intravenous catheter complications, and abnormalities in blood counts and chemistries.

If treatment can be continued long term, then a remarkable degree of recovery is possible. However, attention must be paid to all treatment modalities for such a recovery- not only antibiotics, but rehab and exercise programs, nutritional supplements, enforced rest, low carbohydrate, high fiber diets, attention to food sensitivities, avoidance of stress, abstinence from caffeine and alcohol, and absolutely no immunosuppressants, even local doses of steroids (intra-articular injections, for example).

Unfortunately, not all patients with chronic Lyme disease will fully recover and treatment may not eradicate the active Borrelia infection. Such individuals may have to be maintained on open-ended, ongoing antibiotic therapy, for they repeatedly relapse after antibiotics are stopped. Maintenance antibiotic therapy in this select group is thus mandatory.

In patients who have chronic Lyme, who do not fully respond to antibiotics, one must search for an explanation. In many cases, these patients are found to have pituitary insufficiency of varying degrees. The abnormalities may be extremely subtle, and provocative testing must be done for full diagnosis. Persistent fatigue, limited stamina, hypotension, and loss of libido suggest this possibility.

Similarly, a small but significant number of these patients harbor toxic levels of heavy metals. Challenge testing by knowledgeable, experienced clinicians is necessary for evaluation. Treatment must be directed toward correcting the specific abnormalities found, and post-treatment retesting to assess efficacy of treatment and endpoint of therapy should be done. Suspect this when poor immune responsiveness and persistent neuropathic signs and symptoms are present.

INDICATORS FOR PARENTERAL THERAPY

(The following are guidelines only and are not meant to be absolute. It is based on retrospective study of over 600 patients with late Lyme disease.)

* Illness for greater than one year
* Prior immunosuppressive therapy while infected with Bb.
* Major neurological involvement
* Active synovitis with high sedimentation rate

270

- Elevated protein or cells in the CSF

ADVANCED TREATMENT OPTIONS

PULSE THERAPY consists of administering antibiotics (usually parenteral ones) two to four days in a row per week. This allows for several advantages:
* Dosages are doubled (ie: cefotaxime, 12 g daily), increasing efficacy
* More toxic medications can be used with increased safety (ie: vancomycin)
* May be effective when conventional, daily regimens have failed.
* IV access may be easier or more tolerable
* More agreeable lifestyle for the patient
* Often less costly than daily regimens

Note that this type of treatment is expected to continue for a minimum of ten weeks, and often must continue beyond twenty weeks. The efficacy of this regimen is based on the fact that it takes 48 to 72 hours of continuous bactericidal antibiotic levels to kill the spirochete, yet it will take longer than the four to five days between pulses for the spirochetes to recover. As with all Lyme treatments, specific dosing and scheduling must be tailored to the individual patient's clinical picture based upon the treating physician's best clinical judgment.

COMBINATION THERAPY (see page 12)
This consists of using two or more dissimilar antibiotics simultaneously for antibiotic synergism, to better compensate for differing killing profiles and sites of action of the individual medications, and to cover the three known forms of Bb. A typical combination is the use of a cell wall agent plus a protein inhibitor (ie: amoxicillin plus clarithromycin). Note that GI intolerance and yeast superinfections are the biggest drawbacks to this type of treatment. However, these complications can often be prevented or easily treated, and the clinically observed benefits of this type of regimen clearly have outweighed these problems in selected patients.

LYME DISEASE AND PREGNANCY
It is well known that B. burgdorferi can cross the placenta and infect the fetus. In addition, breast milk from infected mothers has been shown to harbor spirochetes that can be detected by PCR and grown in culture.

The Lyme Disease Foundation in Hartford, CT had kept a pregnancy registry for eleven years beginning in the late 1980s. They found that if patients were maintained on adequate doses of antibiotic therapy during gestation, then no babies were born with Lyme. My own experience over the last twenty years agrees with this.

The options for treating the mother include oral, intramuscular, and intravenous therapy as outlined above. It is vital that peak and trough antibiotic levels be measured if possible at the start of gestation and at least once more during treatment.

During pregnancy, symptoms generally are mild as the hormonal changes seem to mask many symptoms. However, post-partum, mothers have a rough time, with a sudden return of all their Lyme symptoms including profound fatigue. Post partum depression can be particularly severe. I always advise help in the home for at least the first month, so adequate rest and time for needed treatments are assured.

I also advise against breast feeding for obvious reasons as mentioned above.

MONITORING THERAPY
Drug levels are measured, where possible, to confirm adequate dosing. Often, the regimen may have to be modified to optimize the dose. This may have to be repeated again at any time major changes in the treatment regimen occur, and serially during pregnancy. With parenteral therapy, CBC and chem/liver panels are done at least twice each month, especially during symptom flares, with urinalysis and pro-time monitored less frequently.

SAFETY

Over two decades of experience in treating thousands of patients with Lyme has proven that therapy as described above, although intense, is generally well tolerated. The most common adverse reaction seen is allergy to probenecid. In addition, yeast superinfections are seen, but these are generally easily recognized and managed. The induction of Clostridium difficile toxin production is seen most commonly with ceftriaxone, but can occur with any of the antibiotic regimens mentioned in this document. However, pulsed dose therapy and regular use of the lactobacillus preparations seems to be helpful in controlling yeast and antibiotic related colitis, as the number of cases of C. difficile in Lyme patients is low when these guidelines are followed. Be sure to test stool for both toxin A and toxin B when evaluating for C. difficile colitis.

When using central intravenous lines including PICC lines (peripherally inserted central catheters), if ANY line problems arise, it is recommended that the line be pulled for patient safety. Salvage attempts (urokinase, repairing holes) are often ineffective and may not be safe.

Please advise all patients who take the tetracyclines of skin and eye sensitivity to sunlight and the proper precautions, and advise birth control if appropriate. When doxycycline is given parenterally, do not refreeze the solution prior to use!

Remember, years of experience with chronic antibiotic therapy in other conditions, including rheumatic fever, acne, gingivitis, recurrent otitis, recurrent cystitis, COPD, bronchiectasis, and others have not revealed any consistent dire consequences as a result of such medication use. Indeed, the very real consequences of untreated, chronic persistent infection by B. burgdorferi can be far worse than the potential consequences of this treatment.

CO-INFECTIONS IN LYME

PIROPLASMOSIS (Babesiosis)
GENERAL INFORMATION

It had been thought that Babesia microti is the only significant piroplasm affecting humans. Now it is believed that many of the over two dozen known species of piroplasms can be carried by ticks and potentially be transmitted to the human. Unfortunately, we have no widely available tests for these non-microti species. That is why, again, a clinical diagnosis is required.

Piroplasms are not bacteria, they are protozoans. Therefore, they will not be eradicated by any of the currently used Lyme treatment regimens. Therein lies the significance of co-infections- if a Lyme patient has been extensively treated yet is still ill, and especially if they are experiencing atypical symptoms, suspect a co-infection. From the literature:
- "Co-infection generally results in more intense acute illness, a greater array of symptoms, and a more prolonged convalescence than accompany either infection alone."
- "Spirochete DNA was evident more often and remained in the circulation longer in co-infected subjects than in those experiencing either infection alone."
- "Co-infection might also synergize spirochete-induced lesions in human joints, heart and nerves."
- "Babesia infections may impair human host defense mechanisms…"
- "The possibility of concomitant Babesia infection should be considered when moderate to severe Lyme Disease has been diagnosed."

Babesia infection is becoming more commonly recognized, especially in patients who already have Lyme Disease. It has been published that as many as 66% of Lyme patients show serologic evidence of co-infection with Babesia microti. It has also been reported that Babesia infections can range in severity from mild, subclinical infection, to fulminant, potentially life threatening illness. Subclinical infection is often missed because the symptoms are incorrectly ascribed to Lyme. Babesia infections, even mild ones, may recur even after treatment and cause severe illness. This phenomenon has been reported to occur at any time, including up to several years after the initial infection! Furthermore, such Babesia carriers pose a risk to the blood supply as this infection has been reported to be passed on by blood transfusion.

SYMPTOMS
Clues to the presence of Babesiosis include a more acute initial illness- patients often recall a high fever and chills at the onset of their Lyme. Over time, they can note night sweats, air hunger, an occasional cough, persistent migraine-like headache, a vague sense of imbalance without true vertigo, encephalopathy and fatigue. The fulminant presentations are seen in those who are immunosuppressed, especially if asplenic, and in advanced ages. They include high fevers, shaking chills and hemolysis, and can be fatal.

DIAGNOSTIC TESTS
Diagnostic tests are insensitive and problematic. There are at least thirteen, and possibly as many as two dozen Babesia forms found in ticks, yet we can currently only test for B. microti and WA-1 with our serologic and nuclear tests. Standard blood smears reportedly are reliable for only the first two weeks of infection, thus are not useful for diagnosing later infections and milder ones including carrier states where the germ load is too low to be detected. Therefore, multiple diagnostic test methods are available and each have their own benefits and limitations and often several tests must be done. Be prepared to treat based on clinical presentation, even with negative tests.

- SEROLOGY- Unlike Lyme, Babesia titers can reflect infection status. Thus, persistently positive titers or western blots suggest persistent infection.
- PCR- This is more sensitive than smears for B. microti, but will not detect other species.
- ENHANCED SMEAR- This utilizes buffy coat, prolonged scanning (up to three hours per sample!) and digital photography through custom-made microscopes. Although more sensitive than standard smears, infections can still be missed. The big advantage is that it will display multiple species, not just B. microti.
- FLUORESCENT IN-SITU HYBRIDIZATION ASSAY (FISH)- This technique is also a form of blood smear. It is said to be 100-fold more sensitive than standard smears for B. microti, because instead of utilizing standard, ink-based stains, it uses a fluorescent-linked RNA probe and ultraviolet light. The Babesia organisms are then much easier to spot when the slides are scanned. The disadvantage is that currently only B. microti is detected.

TREATMENT
Treating Babesia infections had always been difficult, because the therapy that had been recommended until 1998 consisted of a combination of clindamycin plus quinine. Published reports and clinical experience have shown this regimen to be unacceptable, as nearly half of patients so treated have had to abandon treatment due to serious side effects, many of which were disabling. Furthermore, even in patients who could tolerate these drugs, there was a failure rate approaching 50%.

Because of these dismal statistics, the current regimen of choice for Babesiosis is the combination of atovaquone (Mepron, Malarone), 750 mg bid, plus an erythromycin-type drug, such as azithromycin (Zithromax), clarithromycin (Biaxin), or telithromycin (Ketek) in standard doses. This combination was initially studied in animals, and then applied to Humans with good success. Fewer than 5% of patients have to halt treatment due to side effects, and the success rate is clearly better than that of clindamycin plus quinine.

The duration of treatment with atovaquone combinations for Babesiosis varies depending on the degree of infection, duration of illness before diagnosis, the health and immune status of the patient, and whether the patient is co-infected with Borrelia burgdorferi. Typically, a three-week course is prescribed for acute cases, while chronic, longstanding infections with significant morbidity and co-infection will require a minimum of four months of therapy. Relapses have occurred, and retreatment is occasionally needed.

Problems during therapy include diarrhea, mild nausea, the expense of atovaquone (over $600.00 per bottle-enough for three weeks of treatment), and rarely, a temporary yellowish discoloration of the vision. Blood counts, liver panels and amylase levels are recommended every three weeks during any prolonged course of therapy as liver enzymes may elevate. Treatment failures usually are related to inadequate atovaquone levels. Therefore, patients who are not cured with this regimen can be retreated with higher doses (and atovaquone blood levels can be checked), as this has proven effective in many of my patients. Artemesia (a non-prescription herb) should be added in all cases. Metronidazole or Bactrim can also be added to increase efficacy, but there is minimal clinical data on how much more effective this will be.

BARTONELLA-LIKE ORGANISMS
It has been said that Bartonella is the most common of all tick-borne pathogens. Indeed, there seems to be a fairly distinct clinical syndrome when this type of organism is present in the chronic Lyme patient. However, several aspects of this infection seem to indicate that this tick-associated strain of Bartonella is different from that described as "cat scratch disease". For example, in patients who fit the clinical picture, standard Bartonella blood testing is commonly non-reactive. Furthermore, the usual Bartonella medications do not work for this- they suppress the symptoms but do not permanently clear them. For these reasons I like to refer to this as a "Bartonella-like organism" (BLO), rather than assume it is a more common species.

Indicators of BLO infection include CNS symptoms out of proportion to the other systemic symptoms of chronic Lyme. There seems to be an increased irritability to the CNS, with agitation, anxiety, insomnia, and even seizures, in addition to other unusually strong symptoms of encephalitis, such as cognitive deficits and confusion. Other key symptoms may include gastritis, lower abdominal pain (mesenteric adenitis), sore soles, especially in the AM, tender subcutaneous nodules along the extremities, and red rashes. These rashes may have the appearance of red streaks like stretch marks that do not follow skin planes, spider veins, or red papular eruptions. Lymph nodes may be enlarged and the throat can be sore.

Because standard Bartonella testing, either by serology or PCR, may not pick up this BLO, the blood test is very insensitive. Therefore, the diagnosis is a clinical one, based on the above points. Also, suspect infection with BLO in extensively treated Lyme patients who still are encephalitic, and who never had been treated with a significant course of specific treatment.

The drug of choice to treat BLO is levofloxacin. Levofloxacin is usually never used for Lyme or Babesia, so many patients who have tick-borne diseases, and who have been treated for them but remain ill, may in fact be infected with BLO. Treatment consist of 500 mg daily (may be adjusted based on body weight) for at least one month. Treat for three months or longer in the more ill patient. It has been suggested that levofloxacin may be more effective in treating this infection if a proton pump inhibitor is added in standard doses.

Another subtlety is that certain antibiotic combinations seem to inhibit the action of levofloxacin, while others seem to be neutral. I advise against using an erythromycin-like drug, as clinically such patients do poorly. On the other hand, combinations with cephalosporins, penicillins and tetracyclines are okay. Alternatives to levofloxacin include rifampin, gentamicin and possibly streptomycin. A very recent article suggests that prior use of quinine-like drugs including atovaquone (Mepron, Malarone) may render Levaquin less effective. Therefore, in a co-infected patient, treat the BLO before you address Babesia species.

Levofloxacin is generally well tolerated, with almost no stomach upset. Very rarely, it can cause confusion- this is temporary (clears in a few days) and may be relieved by lowering the dose. There is, however, one side effect that would require it to be stopped- it may cause a painful tendonitis, usually of the largest tendons. If this happens, then the levofloxacin must be stopped or tendon rupture may occur. It has been suggested that loading the patient with magnesium may prevent this problem, and if the tendons do become affected, parenteral high dose vitamin C (plus parenteral magnesium) may afford rapid relief.

Unfortunately, levofloxacin and drugs in this family cannot be given to those under the age of 18, so other alternatives, such as azithromycin, are used in children.

Incidentally, animal studies show that Bartonella may be transmitted across the placenta. No human studies have been done.

EHRLICHIA (AND ANAPLASMA)
GENERAL INFORMATION
While it is true that this illness can have a fulminant presentation, and may even become fatal if not treated, milder forms do exist, as does chronic low-grade infection, especially when other tick-borne organisms are

present. The potential transmission of Ehrlichia during tick bites is the main reason why doxycycline is now the first choice in treating tick bites and early Lyme, before serologies can become positive. When present alone or co-infecting with B. burgdorferi, persistent leukopenia is an important clue. Thrombocytopenia and elevated liver enzymes, common in acute infection, are less often seen in those who are chronically infected, but likewise should not be ignored. Headaches, myalgias, and ongoing fatigue suggest this illness, but are extremely difficult to separate from symptoms caused by Bb.

DIAGNOSTIC TESTING
Testing is problematic with Ehrlichia, similar to the situation with Babesiosis. More species are known to be present in ticks than can be tested for with clinically available serologies and PCRs. In addition, serologies and PCRs are of unknown sensitivity and specificity. Standard blood smears for direct visualization of organisms in leukocytes are of low yield. Enhanced smears using buffy coats significantly raise sensitivity and can detect a wider variety of species. Despite this, infection can be missed, so clinical diagnosis remains the primary diagnostic tool. Again, consider this diagnosis in a Lyme Borreliosis (LB) patient not responding well to Lyme therapy who has symptoms suggestive of Ehrlichia.

TREATMENT
Standard treatment consists of Doxycycline, 200 mg daily for two to four weeks. Higher doses, parenteral therapy, and longer treatment durations may be needed based on the duration and severity of illness, and whether immune defects or extreme age is present. However, there are reports of treatment failure even when higher doses and long duration treatment with doxycycline is given. In such cases, consideration may be given for adding rifampin, 600 mg daily, to the regimen.

SORTING OUT THE CO-INFECTIONS
In addition to *Borrelia burgdorferi* (Bb), ticks may carry and transmit other infections. Furthermore, patients with disseminated Lyme complicated by these co-infections are usually immunocompromized and may also manifest signs and symptoms of reactivated latent infections and opportunists. All can add to morbidity and may need to be treated.

Because of the large number of these other infections, the cost of reliably testing for all of them as a matter of routine is prohibitive. Also, as in the case with Bb infection, laboratory tests for them are often insensitive. Thus there is a need to sort it all out clinically to provide guidance in testing and treatment. Here are some clues:

CLASSIC LYME (Bb infection)-
- Gradual onset of initial (viral-like) symptoms- this often makes it difficult to pinpoint when the infection began.
- Multisystem- almost always, in disseminated stages, involves more than one part or system (i.e. joint pain plus cognitive dysfunction).
- Migratory- first a knee will hurt, then over time this may lessen and the elbow or shoulder acts up, and later the joints calm down but headaches worsen.
- Stiff joints and loud joint crepitus, especially the neck ("Lyme shrug").
- Headaches are often nuchal and associated with stiff, painful and crepitant neck.
- Afternoon fevers, often unnoticed- most Lyme patients have subnormal temperatures in the AM but rise to 99+ by early to mid-afternoon. No obvious sweats.
- Tiredness and limited stamina- often is a strong need to rest or even nap in the afternoon, especially when the flushed face and elevated temperature appears.
- 4-week cycles- Bb activity, and thus symptoms, wax and wane in a cycle that repeats roughly every four weeks. This cycle, if clear, can guide your treatments.
- Slow response to treatment, with an initial symptom flare in most ("Herxheimer-like reaction") then improvement over weeks, punctuated by the monthly symptom flares. Likewise, if treatment is ended too soon, an initial period of well-being will gradually, over a few weeks, be replaced by a return of symptoms.
- EM rash in 25% to 50%

BARTONELLA & "BARTONELLA-LIKE ORGANISMS"-

- Gradual onset of initial illness.
- CNS symptoms are out of proportion to the musculoskeletal ones- if a patient has no or minimal joint complaints but is severely encephalopathic (see below), then think of Bartonella/BLO.
- Obvious signs of CNS irritability can include muscle twitches, tremors, insomnia, seizures, agitation, anxiety, severe mood swings, outbursts and antisocial behavior.
- GI involvement may present as gastritis or abdominal pain (mesenteric adenitis).
- Sore soles, especially in the morning.
- Tender sub-cutaneous nodules along the extremities, especially outer thigh, shins, and occasionally along the triceps.
- Occasional lymphadenopathy.
- Morning fevers, usually around 99. Occasionally light sweats are noted.
- Elevated vascular endothelial growth factor (VEGF) occurs in a minority, but the degree of elevation correlates with activity of the infection and may be used to monitor treatment.
- Rapid response to treatment changes- often symptoms improve within days after antibiotics are begun, but relapses occur also within days if medication is withdrawn early.
- May have papular or linear red rashes (like stretch marks that do not always follow skin planes), especially in those with GI involvement.

BABESIA SPECIES-
- Rapid onset of initial illness, often with sudden onset of high fever, severe headaches, sweats and fatigue, thus it is easy to know when infection began.
- Obvious sweats, usually at night, but can be day sweats as well.
- Air hunger, need to sigh and take a deep breath; dry cough without apparent reason.
- Headaches can be severe - dull, global (involves the whole head, described like the head is in a vise).
- Fatigue is prominent, does not clear with rest, and is made worse with exercise.
- Mental dullness and slowing of reactions and responses.
- Dizziness- more like a tippy feeling, and not vertigo or purely orthostasis.
- Symptoms cycle rapidly, with flares every four to six days.
- Hypercoaguable states are often associated with *Babesia* infections.
- Rarely, splenomegaly
- Very severe Lyme Disease can be a clue to *Babesia* infection, as it will make Lyme symptoms worse and Lyme treatments less effective.

EHRLICHIA/ANAPLASMA-
- Rapid onset of initial illness with fever, headache, prostration.
- Headaches are sharp, knife-like, and often behind the eyes.
- Muscle pain, not joint pain, and can be mild or severe.
- Low WBC count, elevated liver enzymes, and (rarely) inclusions seen in the WBCs.
- Rarely see diffuse vasculitic rash, including palms and soles (less than 10%).
- Rapid response to treatment.

DNA VIRUSES (HHV-6, EBV, CMV)
- Persistent fatigue, made worse with exercise.
- Sore throat, lymphadenopathy, and other viral-like complaints.
- May see elevated liver enzymes and low WBC counts.
- Autonomic dysfunction.

SUPPORTIVE THERAPY

CERTAIN **ABSOLUTE RULES** MUST BE FOLLOWED IF LYME SYMPTOMS ARE TO BE PERMANENTLY CLEARED:
1. Not allowed to get behind in sleep, or become overtired.
2. No caffeine or other stimulants that may affect depth or duration of sleep, or reduce or eliminate naps.

3. Absolutely no alcohol!
4. No smoking at all.
5. Aggressive exercises are required and should be initiated as soon as possible.
6. Diet must contain generous quantities of high quality protein and be high in fiber and low in fat and carbohydrates- no simple carbohydrates are allowed. Instead, use those with low glycemic index.
7. Certain key nutritional supplements should be added.
8. COMPLIANCE!

NUTRITIONAL SUPPLEMENTS IN DISSEMINATED LYME DISEASE

BACKGROUND INFORMATION
Studies on patients with chronic illnesses such as Lyme and Chronic Fatigue have demonstrated that some of the late symptoms are related to cellular damage and deficiencies in certain essential nutrients. Double blinded, placebo controlled studies, and in one case direct assay of biopsy specimens have proven the value of some of the supplements listed. Some are required, while others are optional -see below. They are listed in order of importance.
I suggest patients use a pill organizer. These are multi-compartment boxes that you pre-fill with your pills once a week. This makes the task of taking a large number of tablets much, much simpler and can markedly minimize missed doses. The Vitamin Shop sells a variety of good organizers.

I have found that the quality of supplements used is often more important than the dose. In fact, I do not recommend "mega doses". Instead, seek out, if possible, pharmaceutical grade products, especially if USP certified. I recommend, among others, Pharmanex, Researched Nutritionals and Nature Made products because they fit these criteria. In the list below, it is indicated whether the products should be gotten from Pharmanex, Researched Nutritionals, a different specific manufacturer, or even if a generic substitute is OK.

-To order products from Pharmanex, users need to register as a customer with a referral from another registered customer. You may use my referral number (US9256681) to get started. Call 1-800-487-1000.
-Researched Nutritionals generally markets its products only through physician's offices. If you physician does not do this, he or she can still call the company to order the items for you. The number is 1-800-755-3402.
-Nature Made products are widely available in vitamin stores and pharmacies.

BASIC DAILY REGIMEN (in order of importance)

1. PROBIOTICS (required when on antibiotics)
Kefir: This is a yogurt-like drink that is said to more permanently replenish beneficial flora. It is only necessary to drink 2 to 4 ounces a day.
Acidophilus: the best kinds are frozen or refrigerated to ensure potency. Usual dose is two with each meal. Plan to mix together several different brands to broaden the spectrum. Acidophilus can be gotten from most vitamin stores but some generic brands are of unknown freshness and potency. An alternative that does not need refrigeration and can be taken only once a day is a high potency, patented product called "**Pro Bio**" from Pharmanex. The ultimate mix of pre- and probiotics with soil based organisms is a product called "**Prescript-Assist Pro**" from Researched Nutritionals. This too does not need refrigeration.
In addition, have 4 ounces of sugar-free **yogurt** on occasion.

2. MULTI-VITAMIN (required)
I recommend the **Life Pack** family of multivitamins available through Pharmanex. These are unique supplements- pharmaceutical grade and USP certified, they are the only products clinically proven in double blinded, placebo controlled crossover studies to quench free radicals and raise antioxidant levels in the blood and lipids. Choose LifePak for males under 40, LifePak Women for hormonally active women, LifePak Prenatal when pregnant, and LifePak Prime for postmenopausal women and for men over 40. LifePak Teen is also available. Continue long term.

3. CO-Q10- *required, but do not use while taking the prescription drug atovaquone (Mepron, Malarone).*
Deficiencies have been related to poor function of the heart, limitations of stamina, gum disease, and poor resistance to infections. Heart biopsy studies in Lyme patients indicated that they should take between 300 and 400mg daily. I recommend the Co Q-10 from Researched Nutritionals. One caplet contains 400 mg, so the dose is one a day with food.

4. ALPHA LIPOIC ACID (required)
This facilitates entry of CoQ-10 into mitochondria. Dose is 300 mg twice daily. Generic is OK.

5. VITAMIN B (required).
Clinical studies demonstrated the need for supplemental vitamin B in infections with Borrelia, to help clear neurological symptoms. Take one 50 mg B-complex capsule daily. If neuropathy is severe, an additional 50 mg of B-6 can be added. Generics are OK.

6. MAGNESIUM (required)
Magnesium supplementation is very helpful for the tremors, twitches, cramps, muscle soreness, heart skips and weakness. It may also help in energy level and cognition. The best source is magnesium L-lactate dehydrate ("**Mag-tab SR**", sold by Niche Pharmaceuticals: 1-800-677-0355, and available at Wal-Mart). DO NOT rely on "cal-mag", calcium plus magnesium combination tablets, as they are not well absorbed. Take at least one tablet twice daily. Higher doses increase the benefit and should be tried, but may cause diarrhea. In some cases, intramuscular or intravenous doses may be necessary.

7. ESSENTIAL FATTY ACIDS: (required)
Studies show that when EFAs are taken regularly, statistically significant improvements in fatigue, aches weakness, vertigo, dizziness, memory, concentration and depression are likely. There are two broad classes: GLA (omega-6 oils) and EPA (omega-3 oils), derived respectively from plant and fish oils. This is what to take:
Plant Oil: Use a refrigerated liquid product of mixed omega oils obtained from the local health food store (always avoid capsules as the plant oils within may be rancid and you would never know). Take one to two tablespoons of the liquid oil daily. May be mixed with food, put on salads, etc.
Fish Oil: Use "**Marine Omega**" by Pharmanex. Use four daily, taken on a full stomach (this brand is required because it is made not from fish, but from Krill and is certified to be free of any measurable amounts of heavy metals and organic toxins).

8. NT-FACTOR
This product addresses the mitochondrial damage thought to underlie the metabolic dysfunction associated with chronic diseases which, in patients with tick-borne illnesses, is manifest by fatigue and neurologic dysfunction. *It is the single most reliable agent I have found that can give noticeably increased energy levels.* When supplements known to support neurological function are added (see below), improved cognition and memory often result. Effects will be noted in two to three weeks. It also contains high quality prebiotics and probiotics. Available from Researched Nutritionals.

OPTIONAL SUPPLEMENTS FOR SPECIAL CIRCUMSTANCES

FOR NEUROLOGIC SYMPTOMS- here, the goal is three-fold- supply the metabolic needs, replenish what has become depleted, and protect the neurons and their supportive cells. The "required" supplements, above, must be taken, and the items that follow below are considered "add-ons".

ACETYL-L-CARNITINE- this is taken along with **SAM-e**. This combination can result in noticeable gains in short term memory, mood and cognition. The Acetyl Carnitine also is said to help heart and muscle function. Doses: Acetyl-L-carnitine- 1500-2000 mg daily on empty stomach; SAM-e- 400 mg daily with the acetyl carnitine. Positive results may appear as early as 3 weeks; use for 2 to 3 months, but repeat or extend this course if needed. Available in most vitamin stores; Generic acetyl carnitine is okay, but I recommend "Nature Made" brand SAM-e (also available at most vitamin stores).

METHYLCOBALAMIN (Methyl B12)

Methylcobalamin is a prescription drug derived from vitamin B12. This can help to heal problems with the central and peripheral nervous system, improve depressed immune function, and help to restore more normal sleeping patterns. Many patients note improved energy as well. Because the oral form is not absorbed when swallowed or dissolved under the tongue, Methyl B12 must be taken by injection. Dose is generally 25 mg. (1 c.c.) daily for 3 to 6 months. Long term studies have never demonstrated any side effects from this drug. However, *the urine is expected to turn red shortly after each dose-* if the urine is not red, a higher dose may be needed or the present supply may have lost potency. The injectable form of this is not available in regular drug stores. It must be manufactured (compounded) by specialty pharmacies on order.

GREEN TEA

Green, but not black or white tea contains some of the most potent antioxidants around (80-100 times more effective than vitamin C). I strongly recommend this to any patient with degenerative changes to the central nervous system. At least four cups daily are needed to reap this benefit, and the tea must be decaffeinated. A nice alternative is **"TeGreen"** capsules by Pharmanex. They contain 97% pure tea polyphenols and each capsule is the equivalent of four cups of decaffeinated green tea. Take one to three daily.

CORDYMAX

Cordyceps is a well-known herb from Tibet that has been shown in clinical studies to improve stamina, fatigue, and enhance lung and antioxidant function. It also raises superoxide dismutase levels, important to prevent lesions in the central nervous system, which is why *this (along with green tea) is essential if neurodegeneration is part of your illness.* The positive effects can be dramatic; should be used long term. USP- certified cordyceps is available from Pharmanex as **"CordyMax"**.

CITICHOLINE

Many studies have shown benefits to cognition, *especially memory*. Benefits are slow to notice, so plan to use this long-term. Dose is 500 to 1000 mg twice a day.

FOR IMMUNE SUPPORT
"REISHI MAX "

This enhanced extract from cracked spores of the Reishi mushroom has been shown in clinical studies to augment function of the Natural Killer Cells as well as macrophages. Recommended in all patients who have a CD-57 count below 60. Take four a day. Available only from Pharmanex.

TRANSFER FACTORS are the body's natural signals meant to activate the pathogen-killing effects of the cellular immune system. Therapy with these agents consists of taking both a general stimulator, plus specific transfer factors for the infection you have. Personal experience made me a believer in transfer factor therapy. For Lyme patients, use **Transfer Factor Multi-Immune** as the general stimulant, and **Transfer Factor Lyme-Plus** as the specific agent. Both are exclusives from Researched Nutritionals, and I have found them to be surprisingly effective in making the very ill respond better to treatment. Take as directed on the label.

FOR JOINT SYMPTOMS
GLUCOSAMINE

Glucosamine can be of long term benefit to the joints. Do not be misled into buying a product that also contains chondroitin, as this chemical does not add anything, but it can make the product more expensive. Look for a product that contains the herb Boswellia serrata- this is a non-irritative anti-inflammatory. Although many generics exist, the Pharmanex product, **"Cartilage Formula"** has the right ingredients and is of proven efficacy. Expect improvement only over time (several weeks), but plan to use this indefinitely to maintain joint health.

VITAMIN C

Vitamin C is important to aid in maintaining healthy connective tissues. High doses are recommended- 1000 to 6000 mg a day as tolerated (if the dose is too high for you it may cause acid stomach, gas and loose stools, so therefore dose titration is necessary). Consider using **"Ester-C"** (non-acid and longer acting), or **"C-Salts"** (very well tolerated). Start with a low dose and increase slowly to find your tolerance level.

FLEX CREAM
This is an amazing liniment-like product that really works and has a money back guarantee. Use for any type of body pain- spread on a thick layer and do not rub in. It takes 30 to 60 minutes to work, then lasts many hours. A Pharmanex exclusive.

OTHER OPTIONAL SUPPLEMENTS
VITAMIN D
Surprisingly, most people in America are vitamin D deficient. In the Lyme patient, low vitamin D levels can cause diffuse body aches and cramps that are not responsive to magnesium or calcium supplements. Some also believe that vitamin D is essential for normal immune and hormone function. I strongly urge you to have a fasting blood level drawn. It is recommended that the blood levels be in the upper half or the normal range. If it is not, then 2000 to 4000 units daily are needed for several weeks to make up for the deficit, and then a lower maintenance dose may be necessary, based on results from repeated blood level monitoring. If vitamin D is needed, improvements take 2 to 3 weeks to note, but are well worth the wait.

CREATINE
Creatine has been shown to be of benefit in neuromuscular degenerative diseases such as Lou Gherig's Disease (ALS) and can be very helpful in supporting low blood pressure, as in NMH. It may also benefit strength, stamina, and heart function. Important: To use this safely, you must have an adequate fluid intake. The creatine product should contain taurine, an amino acid needed to enhance creatine absorption, plus some carbohydrate to aid creatine entry into muscle. You will need a 20 gram daily loading dose for the first five days, then 4 to 10 grams daily maintenance. Try **"Cell Tech"** from the Vitamin Shop, and follow label directions.

MILK THISTLE
Useful to support liver function. Take 175 mg daily- use an 80% Silymarin extract. Available from many vitamin stores.

LYME DISEASE REHABILITATION

Despite antibiotic treatments, patients will NOT return to normal unless they exercise, so therefore an aggressive rehab program is absolutely necessary. It is a fact that a properly executed exercise program can actually go beyond the antibiotics in helping to clear the symptoms and to maintain a remission.

Although the scientific basis for the benefits of exercises is not known, there are several reasonable theories. It is known that Bb will die if exposed to all but the tiniest oxygen concentrations. If an aggressive exercise program can increase tissue perfusion and oxygen levels, then this may play a role in what is being seen. Also, during aggressive exercise, the core body temperature can rise above 102 degrees; it is known that B. burgdorferi is very heat sensitive. Perhaps it is the added tissue oxygenation, or higher body temperature, or the combination that weakens the Lyme Borrelia, and allows the antibiotics and our defenses to be more effective. Regular exercise-related movements can help mobilize lymph and enhance circulation. In addition, there is now evidence that a carefully structured exercise program may benefit T-cell function: this function will depress for 12 to 24+ hours after exercise, but then rebound. This T-cell depression is more pronounced after aerobics which is why aerobics are not allowed. The goal is to exercise intermittently, with exercise days separated by days of total rest, including an effort to have plenty of quality sleep. The trick is to time the exercise days to take advantage of these rebounds. For an example, begin with an exercise day followed by 3 to 5 rest days; as stamina improves, then fewer rest days will be needed in between workouts. However, because T-cell functions do fall for at least one day after aggressive exercises, be sure to never exercise two days in a row. Finally, an in intermittent exercise program, properly executed, may help to reset the HPA axis more towards normal. On the following page is an exercise prescription that details these recommendations.

This program may begin with classical physical therapy if necessary. The physical therapy should involve massage, heat, ultrasound and simple range of motion exercises to relieve discomfort and promote better sleep and flexibility. Ice (vasoconstriction) and electrical stimulation (muscle spasm and trauma) should not be used!

The program must evolve into a graded, ultimately strenuous exercise program that consists of a specific regimen of *non-aerobic* conditioning- see below. Have the patient complete a gentle hour of prescribed exercise, then go home, have a hot bath or shower, than try to take a nap. Initially, patients will need this sleep, but as they recover, the exercise will energize them and then a nap will no longer be needed. NOTE: a cardiac stress test may be necessary prior to exercising to ensure safety.

LYME REHAB-PHYSICAL THERAPY PRESCRIPTION

NAME_____

D.O.B._____ DATE_____

Please enroll this patient in a program of therapy to rehabilitate him/her from the effects of chronic tick-borne diseases. If necessary, begin with classic physical therapy, then progress when appropriate to a **whole body conditioning program.**

THERAPEUTIC GOALS (to be achieved <u>in order</u> as the patient's ability allows):

<u>PHYSICAL THERAPY</u> (if needed):
1. **The role of physical therapy here is to prepare the patient for the required, preferably gym-based exercise program outlined below. Plan on several weeks of classic PT then transition to the gym.**
2. Relieve pain and muscle spasms utilizing multiple modalities as available and as indicated: massage, heat, ultrasound, and passive and active range of motion. DO NOT use ice or electrical stim unless specifically ordered by our office. Paraffin baths can be quite useful.
3. Increase mobility, tone and strength while protecting damaged and weakened joints, tendons, and ligaments, and teach these techniques to the patient. Use minimal resistance but a lot of repetitions in any exercises prescribed. At the start of the exercise program, especially if the patient is weak, avoid free weights, bands and large exercise balls, and favor machines (especially hydraulics) that can guide limbs through a prescribed arc; free weights, etc. can risk hyperextension and uncontrolled movements that may cause or add to injuries. Transition the patient slowly to the gym-based program outlined below. **Note- aerobics are not permitted.**
4. Please see the patient two or three days per week- but do not schedule two days in a row!

<u>EXERCISE</u> Begin with a private trainer for careful direction and education.

PATIENT EDUCATION AND MANAGEMENT (to be done during the initial one-on-one sessions and reinforced at all visits thereafter):
1. Instruct patients on **correct exercise technique**, including proper warm-up, breathing, joint protection, proper body positioning during the exercise, and how to cool-down and stretch afterwards.
2. Please work one muscle group at a time and perform extensive and extended **stretching** to each muscle group immediately after each one is exercised, before moving on to the next muscle group.
3. A careful **interview** should be performed at the start of each session to make apparent the effects, both good and bad, from the prior visit's therapy, and adjust therapy accordingly.

PROGRAM:
1. **Aerobic exercises are NOT allowed**, not even low impact variety, until the patient has recovered.
2. **Conditioning**: work to improve strength and reverse the poor conditioning that results from Lyme, through a whole-body exercise program, consisting of light calisthenics and/or resistance training, using light resistance and many repetitions. This can be accomplished in exercise classes called "stretch and tone", or "body sculpture", or can be achieved in the gym with exercise machines or carefully with free weights (see cautions above).
3. **Each session should last one hour**. A gentle hour is preferable to a strenuous half-hour. If the patient is unable to continue for the whole hour, then decrease the intensity to allow him/her to do so.
4. **Exercise no more often than every other day**. The patient may need to start by exercising every 4th or 5th day initially, and as abilities improve, work out more often, but NEVER two days in a row. The non-exercise days should be spent resting.
5. This whole-body conditioning program is what is required to achieve wellness. A simple walking program will not work, and simply placing the patient on a treadmill or an exercise bike is not acceptable (except very briefly, as part of a warm-up), as aerobics can be damaging and must be avoided.

PHYSICIAN'S SIGNATURE_____

MANAGING YEAST OVERGROWTH

Many patients with weakened defenses, such as from chronic illnesses, including Lyme Disease, develop an overgrowth of yeast. This begins in the mouth and then spreads to the intestinal tract. Therefore the primary line of defense is careful oral hygiene, replenishing the beneficial bacteria by daily intake of yogurt, Kefir, and/or acidophilus, and by following a strict low carbohydrate diet.

ORAL HYGEINE:

CLEANSING

Brush the teeth, tongue, gums, inner cheeks and palate first with toothpaste, then again for 30 seconds while holding an antiseptic mouthwash in the mouth Then, rinse by scrubbing while holding plain water in the mouth.

TOOTHPASTE

Use "AP-24" toothpaste, sold by NuSkin Enterprises. Unlike conventional toothpastes that may contain alcohols, formaldehydes and abrasives, this product cleans in a unique way. It contains two "surfactants" (detergent-like cleansers) that are very effective without being harsh. This product is available in two forms- regular and whitening (both contain fluoride). Choose either one.

In addition, get from them their patented toothbrush that is designed to work with this toothpaste. It cleans better and is far gentler than regular or electric toothbrushes.

Order AP-24 products by calling 1-800-487-1000. The U.S. reference # is 9256681-R

MOUTHWASHES

Use an antiseptic mouthwash (Scope, Listerine, etc.), and brush the teeth, tongue, gums, cheeks and the roof of the mouth while holding the mouthwash in the mouth. Do this for 30 seconds, then rinse repeatedly with water.

For especially thick or resistant thrush, the most effective (and drastic) treatment, employed as a last resort, consists of using "Dakin's Solution" as a mouth rinse. Make this by mixing one teaspoon of household liquid bleach (Clorox) in four ounces of water. A small amount is held in the mouth while brushing, then spit out, and repeated until the thrush has cleared. This is usually a one-time treatment, but may have to be repeated every few weeks.

After using an antiseptic, it is necessary to immediately eat yogurt or chew an acidophilus capsule to replenish the beneficial flora in the mouth. Because the germ count, both harmful and beneficial, will be artificially reduced after such a cleaning, and because yeasts are opportunists, the yeast infection can come back. By having the yogurt or acidophilus then, the yeast will be crowded out and a more normal oral flora will result.

INTESTINAL TRACT: An overgrowth of yeast here will ferment dietary sugars and starches, forming acids, gas, alcohols and a variety of organic chemicals. Symptoms include gas, bloat, heartburn and/or pain in the stomach area, and because of the organic chemicals, there can be headaches, dizziness, lightheadedness, wooziness and post-meal fatigue. To clear intestinal yeast, first the tongue and mouth must be cleansed so yeast does not reenter the system with every swallow. Next, since yeast germs feed on sugars and starches, follow the low carbohydrate diet outlined below. Finally, to replenish the normal, beneficial microbes, eat PLAIN yogurt daily, drink Kefir, 4 ounces daily, and/or take acidophilus, 2 capsules three times daily after meals.

YEAST CONTROL DIET- restricted carbohydrate regimen

UNRESTRICTED FOODS

All protein foods, such as meat, fish, fowl, cheese, eggs, dairy, tofu

RESTRICTED FOODS
FRUITS

Fruits may be a problem because they contain a large amount of sugars. However, if the fruit contains a lot of fiber, this may make up for the sugars to some degree. Thus:

- Fruits are only allowed at the end of a meal, and never on an empty stomach
- Only high fiber fruits are allowed
- Only very small amounts!

EXAMPLES:
ALLOWED IN GENEROUS AMOUNTS
Grapefruit, lemons, limes, tomatoes, avocado
ALLOWED IN SMALL AMOUNTS ONLY! (The high fiber content in these hard, crunchy fruits partially
    makes up for the carbohydrates)
    Pears, apples, strawberries, cantaloupe, etc.
NOT ALLOWED (These soft fruits do not have enough fiber)
Oranges, watermelons, bananas, grapes, etc.
No fruit juices either!

VEGETABLES
Green vegetables and salads are O.K. Avoid or limit starchy vegetables (potato, rice, beans, etc.) and avoid
pasta.

STARCHES
None!! If it is made from flour- any kind of flour- it is not allowed. (No breads, cereals, cake, pasta, etc.)

SWEETENERS
NOT ALLOWED
No sugars at all, and no fructose or corn syrup
ALLOWED (if tolerated)
Stevia (safest), honey, and Splenda (if tolerated)
Aspartame (NutraSweet, Equal) may not be tolerated by some patients
Saccharin products are not recommended

DRINKS
ALLOWED
Water, seltzer, caffeine-free diet sodas, coffee and tea without sugar or caffeine, vegetable juices
NOT ALLOWED
Fruit juices, regular sodas, and any drinks sweetened with sugars or syrups
No Alcohol at all

OTHERS
Do not skip any meals. At least three regular meals daily are needed; a better option is to eat very small
portions but have between meal snacks to maintain blood sugar and insulin levels. Bedtime snacks, if taken,
must be totally carbohydrate free!

PATIENT INSTRUCTIONS ON TICK BITE PREVENTION AND TICK REMOVAL

HOW TO PROTECT YOURSELF FROM TICK BITES

PROPERTY Remove wood piles, rock walls, and bird feeders as these attract tick-carrying small animals and can increase the risk of acquiring Lyme.
INSECTICIDES: Property should be treated with a product designed to target the rodents that carry ticks- bait boxes and a product called "Damminix" can be used. Use these products in conjunction with liquid or granular insecticides.
LIQUID & GRANULAR PESTICIDES: Products meant for widespread application such as permethrin and its derivatives are preferred. They are available as a liquid concentrate and as granules. If liquid insecticides are used, application should be by fogging, not by coarse sprays. Apply these products in a strip a few feet wide at the perimeter of the lawn at any areas adjacent to woods and underbrush. Also treat any ornamental shrubs near the house that may serve as a habitat for small animals. The best time to apply these products is in late Spring and early Fall. In every case, professional application is recommended.

CLOTHING When wearing long pants, tuck the cuffs into the socks so any ticks that get on shoes or socks will crawl on the outside of the pants and be less likely to bite. Also, light colored clothing should be worn so the ticks will be easier to spot. Smooth materials such as windbreakers are harder for ticks to grab onto and are preferable to knits, etc.

Tick repellents that contain "permethrin" (Permanone, Permakill) are meant to be sprayed onto clothing. Spray the clothes before they're put on, and let them dry first. Do not apply this chemical directly to the skin.

Ticks are very intolerant of being dried out. After being outdoors in an infested area, place clothes in the dryer for a few minutes to kill any ticks that may still be present.

SKIN: Insect repellents that contain "DEET" are somewhat effective when applied to the arms, legs, and around the neck. Do not use any repellent over wide areas of the body as they can be absorbed causing toxicity. Also, it is inadvisable to use a product that contains more than 50% DEET, and 25% concentrations are preferred. Use repellents cautiously on small children, as they are more susceptible to their toxic effects. Be aware that this repellent evaporates quickly and must be reapplied frequently.

Check carefully for ticks not only when you get home but frequently while still outside!

HOW TO REMOVE AN ATTACHED TICK
Using a tweezer (not fingers!), grasp the tick as close to the skin as possible and pull straight out. Then apply an antiseptic. Do not try to irritate them with heat or chemicals, or grasp them by the body, as this may cause the tick to inject <u>more</u> germs into your skin. Tape the tick to a card and record the date and location of the bite. Remember, the sooner the tick is removed, the less likely an infection will result.

APPENDIX
RATIONALE FOR TREATING TICK BITES
Prophylactic antibiotic treatment upon a known tick bite is recommended for those who fit the following categories:
1. People at higher health risk bitten by an unknown type of tick or tick capable of transmitting Borrelia burgdorferi, e.g., pregnant women, babies and young children, people with serious health problems, and those who are immunodeficient.
2. Persons bitten in an area highly endemic for Lyme Borreliosis by an unidentified tick or tick capable of transmitting B. burgdorferi.
3. Persons bitten by a tick capable of transmitting B. burgdorferi, where the tick is engorged, or the attachment duration of the tick is greater than four hours, and/or the tick was improperly removed. This means when the body of the tick is squeezed upon removal, irritated with toxic chemicals in an effort to get it to back out, or disrupted in such a way that its contents were allowed to contact the bite wound. Such practices increase the risk of disease transmission.

4. A patient, when bitten by a known tick, clearly requests oral prophylaxis and understands the risks. This is a case-by-case decision.

The physician cannot rely on a laboratory test or clinical finding at the time of the bite to definitely rule in or rule out Lyme Disease infection, so must use clinical judgment as to whether to use antibiotic prophylaxis. Testing the tick itself for the presence of the spirochete, even with PCR technology, is helpful but not 100% reliable.

An established infection by B. burgdorferi can have serious, long-standing or permanent, and painful medical consequences, and be expensive to treat. Since the likelihood of harm arising from prophylactically applied anti-spirochetal antibiotics is low, and since treatment is inexpensive and painless, it follows that the risk-benefit ratio favors tick bite prophylaxis.

SUGGESTED ADDITIONAL READING

Evidence Based Guidelines for the Management of Lyme Disease. The International Lyme and Associated Diseases Society. Expert Rev. Anti-infect. Ther.2(1), Suppl. (2004)

Lyme Disease: Point/Counterpoint. Stricker, Raphael B. Lautin, Andrew. Burrascano, Joseph J. Expert Rev. Anti-infect. Ther, April 2005. 3(2), 155-165

An Understanding of Laboratory Testing for Lyme Disease. Harris, Nick S. J. Spiro. and Tick-Borne Dis. Vol 5, 1998. 16-26

Gestational Lyme Borreliosis. MacDonald, Alan B. Rheumatic Diseases Clinics of North America 15 (4), Nov. 1989. 657-678

Cerebral Malaria. Newton, Charles R.et al. J. Neurol. Neurosurg. Psychiatry. 2000. Vol 69, 433-441.

RESOURCES

International Lyme and Associated Diseases Society
www.ILADS.org
P.O. Box 341461
Bethesda, MD 20827-1461

Lyme Disease Association, Inc.
P.O. Box 1438, Jackson, NJ 08527
(888) 366-6611
www.lymediseaseassociation.org

286

APPENDIX B

Healthy Fats to Take With Mepron and Malarone

Mepron and Malarone are special cases as they absorb best when taken with fatty food. But before you rush out for a helping of French fries, think first of the healthy ways you can get those fats!

Research shows that 20-25 grams of fat is ideal; absorption studies have been done using 23 grams. Here are some amounts of fat contained in various foods.

Eggs	1 medium	5 grams
Cashew/ almond butter	1 tablespoon	10 grams
Tahini (sesame butter)	1 tablespoon	8 grams
Avocado	1 medium	30 grams
Coconut oil	1 tablespoon	14 grams
Kefir	1 cup (250ml)	8.75 grams
Almonds (raw)	1/4 cup	11.5 grams
Chicken breast	single (1/2 breast)	3.2 grams
Sausage (pork)	1 link	7 grams
Sausage (chicken)	1 link	10 grams
Cheese (cheddar)	1 oz slice	9 grams

Fat content of fish and flax oil supplements

Omega-3 supplements are definitely healthy fats but in gel cap form will not meet the amount of fat required for the absorption of Mepron. Fatty acids in liquid form are better bets.

Fish oil (gel caps)	1 gel cap	5 grams
Fish oil (liquid)	1 tablespoon	15 grams
Flax oil (Omega Swirl)	1 tablespoon	5 grams
Flax oil (liquid)	1 tablespoon	15 grams

So, here are some suggestions for what to eat along with each dose of Mepron:

- 2 ½ tablespoons cashew or almond butter
- 1 ½ tablespoons coconut oil
- 1 ¼ tablespoons fish or flax oil
- 4 tablespoons Omega Swirl
- 2 ½ tablespoons tahini
- ½ cup almonds
- 3 large eggs

APPENDIX C

Summary of Medications and Common Dosages

Form of Borrelia	Medication Class	Commonly Used Examples
Spirochetes	Penicillins	Amoxicillin, Bicillin LA
	Cephalosporins	Cefuroxime, Ceftriaxone
Cell-wall deficient	Macrolides	Azithromycin, Clarithromycin
	Tetracyclines	Doxycycine, Minocycline
Cyst forms		Tinidazole, Metronidazole
		Hydroxychloroquine
		(Plaquenil), Alinia

The ultimate goal of therapy for Borrelia:

- 1 cell-wall active medication (for spirochetes)
- 2 intracellular medications (for cell-wall deficient forms)
- 1 cyst form medication (for cysts)

Plus medications added for relevant co-infections.

Common Dosages

Penicillins:

• Amoxicillin	1000mg	3-6 daily
• Augmentin XR	2000mg	2x daily
• Bicillin LA	1.2 mill	1 vial injected IM 3x weekly

Cephalosporins:

• Cefuroxime	500mg	3x daily
• Ceftriaxone	2 gram	2 grams twice daily IV 4days/week
• Cefdinir	300mg	2x daily

Macrolides:

• Azithromycin	500mg	1x daily
• Clarithromycin	500mg	2x daily
• Telithromycin	800mg	1x daily

Tetracyclines:

• Minocycline	100mg	3-4x daily
• Doxycycline	100mg	2 twice daily
• Tetracycline	500mg	3-4x daily

Cyst-form medications:

• Metronidazole	500mg	2x daily; 2 weeks on/ 2 weeks off
• Tinidazole	500mg	2x daily; 2 weeks on/ 2 weeks off
• Plaquenil	200mg	2x daily

Babesia medications:

• Mepron	750mg/ 5mL	1-2 teaspoons twice daily
• Malarone	250/ 100mg	2 twice daily
• Lariam	250mg	1 every five days
• Alinia	500mg	2x daily

Bartonella, Ehrlichia, Anaplasma, Rickettsia medications:

• Rifampin	300mg	2x daily
• Levaquin	500mg	1x daily
• Bactrim DS	800/160mg	2x daily

APPENDIX D

Coping With Herx Reactions

A Herx reaction is caused by neurotoxins released by microbes when they are being killed off. A Herx usually starts a few days into treatment—starting a new medication or supplement that is killing bugs. Herx reactions can last anywhere from a few hours to days or even weeks.

To minimize Herx reactions here are some things that can be helpful:

- Drink fresh squeezed lemon or lime juice in warm water, 2-3 times daily. Clean your teeth afterwards to protect tooth enamel, as lemon and lime juice are acidic.
- Drink ionized, alkaline water – 2 liters per day.
- Eat a clean diet of lean proteins, healthy uncooked oils and vegetables. Juice greens if possible or drink wheat grass juice.
- Take Epsom salts baths as the magnesium sulfate assists with detox. Magnesium is also relaxing for sore aching muscles.
- Alka-Seltzer Gold (must be gold, not regular) can be helpful.
- Try to rest and sleep as much as possible.
- Use far infrared sauna if possible, but only for short durations as tolerated.
- Do coffee enemas to help the liver and bowels flush out toxin

Supplements to take or increase during a Herx:

- Dr Nicola's Smilax – this herbal tincture helps to neutralize neurotoxins. 1-2 droppersful twice daily in water.

- Dr Nicola's Detox Formula (#1 or #2) – herbs to assist the function of the liver and to cleanse the blood. 1-2 droppersful twice daily in water.
- TriFortify Liposomal Glutathione – 1 teaspoon in water once or twice daily.
- Dr Nicola's Nerve Pain Formula – for symptomatic relief of nerve pain such as burning and stabbing pain, and headache/ migraine.
- Activated Charcoal – 1-2 capsules twice daily 2 hours apart from other meds/ supplements. Acts as a binding agent in the gut to bind up the neurotoxins.
- Fiber blend containing soluble and insoluble fiber (such as Dr. Nicola's Fiber Plus) – to help bind and sweep out bowels to get toxins out.

APPENDIX E

Castor Oil Pack Instructions

Castor oil packs aid in elimination and detoxification processes in the body and have been used for a variety of conditions ranging from chole-cystitis (inflammation of the gall bladder) to sluggish liver, poor elimination, headaches and toxemia.

A castor oil pack is an external application of castor oil. A piece of wool flannel is saturated in castor oil and applied to the upper right quadrant of the abdomen (over the liver) with a heating pad. The purpose is to increase detoxification via the liver and lymphatic system, to reduce inflammation through cytokine modulation, and to improve the function of the colon. This can have a positive impact on systemic inflammation improving symptoms such as joint pain, headache, constipation and abdominal pain.

Castor oil packs should be used with caution or avoided if one has bleeding disorders and active ulcers, or is pregnant. Individuals with chemical sensitivity disorders may have an increase in symptoms after using the castor oil pack, especially at the beginning of treatment, as it aids (and stimulates) the process of elimination and detoxification. Initially, it may be best to shorten the length of time of the castor oil pack treatment.

What You Will Need

- Flannel Cloth (cotton or wool, washed and dried, 20" to 40" x 24" to 48")
- Plastic wrap (clear kitchen plastic wrap or plastic bag without printing)
- Glass dish (Pyrex or similar dish large enough to warm the flannel castor oil pack prior to use)
- Old bath towel
- Hot water bottle or hot gel pack
- Castor oil
- Large zip-lock bag

Directions

1. Fold the washed and dried flannel cloth so that it is 2-3 layers thick and fits over most of your abdomen.
2. Soak the flannel cloth in castor oil. Strip or loosely wring out the excess oil. There will be excess oil for the first few applications. After that the castor oil pack should not drip excess oil.
3. Put the castor oil pack in a heat-safe glass dish and place in the oven or in the microwave to heat to a comfortable temperature.
4. Lie down in a comfortable position. You may want to place a plastic sheet or an old towel under you during the initial applications to avoid oil stains from getting on your bedding, upholstery or carpeting. Place the castor oil pack directly on your abdomen.
5. Cover the pack with a sheet of plastic, again to avoid staining.
6. Wrap an old towel around your abdomen to hold the castor oil pack in place and secure. Place a hot water bottle or gel pack over the towel. Wrap yourself in a warm blanket.
7. Leave the castor oil pack on for 45-60 minutes or overnight.
8. It is fine to fall asleep with the castor oil pack on, as long as you are not using an electrical heating source.
9. When you are done, store the pack in a large zip-lock bag in the refrigerator. The pack can be used repeatedly, adding more castor oil as needed. The castor oil pack can be used for several months.

APPENDIX F

Dry Skin Brushing Instructions

The skin is the largest organ of the body and is responsible for a significant amount of the body's elimination processes (approximately one quarter each day). The skin and the lungs are often forgotten when we discuss detoxification, with the liver and kidneys receiving most of the attention. Granted, most medications clear through the liver and/or kidneys, however the skin, with its porous structure and vast surface area, should not be forgotten.

Skin brushing is a technique that assists in clearing the lymphatic system, improving the surface circulation on the skin, keeping the pores opens, encouraging the body's discharge of metabolic wastes, and boosting immune function. The lymphatic system is the waste management system of the body, transporting the waste products that have been filtered from the blood back to the large vessels for proper excretion. The lymph system often gets sluggish and backed up with wastes, so clearing it is important.

Benefits of skin brushing:

- Tightens skin
- Removes dead skin cells
- "Sweeps" the lymphatic fluid back towards the heart for proper elimination
- Encourages healthy cell renewal and exchange of wastes and nutrients between cells

- Strengthens the immune system
- Stimulates the glands, encouraging optimal function

The key to effective skin brushing is selecting the right brush. The brush should have natural fibers, not synthetic, as synthetic bristles will scratch the skin and create irritation. Natural fibers should feel soft on the skin. At first the skin may feel a little itchy after brushing as the circulation is stimulated, but this will subside after the first few times. I like the boar hairbrushes by Bass. They are available online or in many health food stores. Purchase one with a long handle so you can brush all parts of your body, even your back and legs.

The second key is brushing towards the heart. Imagine that your lymphatic system is carrying waste material towards the heart to dump into the large veins of the body. We are trying to assist by "sweeping" that material towards the heart, so always use strokes that go in one direction only, towards the heart. The only exception to this is around the chest area itself, where you can brush towards the armpits.

The third key is always brushing dry skin, before a shower is ideal as then you rinse away any dead skin cells that you have sloughed during brushing. Brushing wet skin will not have the same effect. Try to brush once or twice daily.

APPENDIX G

Summary of Biofilm Protocols

Biofilm protocols have five main goals:

1. Eat through the goo-like matrix using enzymes and thinning agents
2. Break the bonds between the goo using Ca-EDTA
3. Kill the now-exposed bugs using antimicrobials
4. Sweep the whole mess out using fibers and binders
5. Rebuild the gut lining with happy, healthy critters

Breaking Down the Biofilm Structure

Boulouke Lumbrokinase – this is a substance that acts as a fibrinolytic and anti-coagulant agent. In other words, it can thin out blood that is too thick and "sticky", and reduce the density of the biofilm. 1-2 capsules 30 minutes before meals, 3x daily.

InflaQuell – these are proteolytic enzymes that were discussed under the anti-inflammatory category. Because of their ability to break down proteins they are also useful in breaking down the biofilm matrix. 3 capsules twice daily on an empty stomach.

Breaking Bonds Between the Goo Structure

Ca-EDTA has classically been used as a heavy metal chelator with an affinity for lead. In the context of biofilm, it can be effective in complexing with the ions that hold the matrix together, thus reducing the ability of the matrix to hold together.

Killing the Bugs that are Now Exposed and Not Hiding/Stuck in the Goo

This can be antibiotics, natural antimicrobials, or a combination of both. Care must be taken as killing these newly exposed bugs can cause a Herx.

Sweeping Out the Residues

(both the polysaccharide matrix residues and the die-off products from the bugs themselves)

Toxi HMF (BioGenesis) is a good option for this as it contains apple pectin, sodium alginate and bentonite clay which all serve to bind and facilitate excretion. Psyllium husk and ground up flax seeds in a 1:4 ratio also accelerate this process. This mix can be blended into a smoothie or mixed with kefir. If a lot of endotoxins have been released, then cholestyramine may be a good option, but that can bind with many medications and supplements so care must be taken with timing.

Rebuilding the Gut Lining

Emphasis on probiotics such as Prescript-Assist Pro to recolonize the gut with healthy flora. Sometimes intensive recolonization with high potency products such as RestorProbiotic Powder may be needed (these two contain upwards of 100 billion organisms per dose.

APPENDIX H

Sample Naturopathic Protocols

* RestorMedicine products

** Researched Nutritionals

More information and ordering at www.restormedicine.com.

Detoxification Support

- Smilax *   40 drops twice daily
- Detox Support Formula *   40 drops twice daily
- Tri-Fortify Glutathione **   1 teaspoon in the morning in water
- Dr. Nicola's Detox Plus Powder * 2 scoops daily

Immune Support

- Transfer Factor Multi-Immune **   2 capsules before bed
- Transfer Factor LymPlus **   2 capsules before bed

Digestive Support

- RestorProbiotic Powder *   ½ - 1 scoop before bed
- (or) Prescript Assist **   2 capsules at night before bed
- Dr. Nicola's Fiber Plus *   4 capsules at night
- Anti-Parasite Formula *   40 drops three times daily
- Anti-Fungal Formula *   40 drops three times daily

Pain and Inflammation

- Soothe and Relaxx **   3 capsules twice daily
- InflaQuell **   3 capsules twice daily between meals
- Nerve Pain Formula *   40 drops three or four times daily

Mood and Sleep

- Soothe and Relaxx **   3 capsules twice daily
- Dr. Nicola's Sleep Support *   2 to 4 capsules before bed
- 200mg of Zen (ARG)   2 capsules twice daily
- 5-HTP   50mg   1 twice daily for mood; up to 4 before bed for sleep

Cognitive Function

- Tri-Fortify Glutathione **   1 teaspoon in the morning in water
- Cognicare **   2 twice daily

Adrenal Support (Energy)

- Energy Multiplex **   3 capsules in the morning
- Licorice Plus (Metagenics)   2 tablets twice daily
- Adreset (Metagenics)   1 capsule twice daily
- DHEA Plus (Douglas Labs)   1 capsule daily in the morning

Mitochondrial Support (Energy)

- ATP Fuel **   5 capsules twice daily
- CoQ10 400mg **   1 capsule daily
- Ribos-Cardio **   1 scoop daily

Antimicrobial

- Teasel Root *   5 drops twice daily
- Lyme Support Formula *   10 drops twice daily
- Artemisinin SOD **   2 capsules twice daily
- HH2 Formula (Zhang)   1 capsule three times daily

Biofilm

- Boulouke Lumbrokinase **   1 capsule twice daily between meals
- InflaQuell **   3 capsules twice daily between meals
- Interfase Plus (Klaire Labs)   2 capsules twice daily between meals

Heavy Metal Chelation

- Chelex (Xymogen)   4 capsules one or two times daily
- DMSA 250mg (Thorne)   1 capsule three times daily, 3 days on/ 7 days off
- EDTA 750mg (compounded)   1 suppository every other night
- Multiple Mineral (Klaire Labs) 2 capsules on non-DMSA/ non-EDTA days

The Top 10 Lyme Disease Treatments: Defeat Lyme Disease With The Best Of Conventional And Alternative Medicine

By Bryan Rosner
Foreword by James Schaller, M.D.

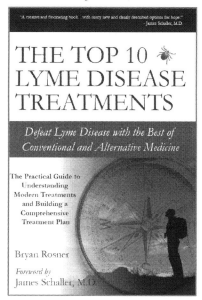

"A creative and fascinating book...with many new and clearly described options for hope."
- James Schaller, M.D.

THE TOP 10
LYME DISEASE
TREATMENTS

Defeat Lyme Disease with the Best of Conventional and Alternative Medicine

The Practical Guide to Understanding Modern Treatments and Building a Comprehensive Treatment Plan

Bryan Rosner
Foreword by
James Schaller, M.D.

Book • $35

This information-packed book identifies ten promising conventional and alternative Lyme disease treatments and gives practical guidance on integrating them into a comprehensive treatment plan that you and your physician can customize for your individual situation and needs.

The book was not written to replace Bryan Rosner's first book (*Lyme Disease and Rife Machines*, opposing page). It was written to complement that book, offering Lyme sufferers many new foundational and supportive treatment options, based on the author's extensive research and years of personal experience. Topics include*:

- Systemic enzyme therapy, which helps detoxify tissues and blood, reduce inflammation, stimulate the immune system, and kill Lyme disease bacteria.
- Lithium orotate, a powerful yet all-natural mineral (belonging to the same mineral group as sodium and potassium) capable of profound neuroprotective activity.
- Thorough and extensive coverage of a complete Lyme disease detoxification program, including discussion of both liver and skin detoxification pathways. Specific detoxification therapies such as liver cleanses, bowel cleanses, the Shoemaker Neurotoxin Elimination Protocol, sauna therapy, mineral baths, mineral supplementation, milk thistle, and many others. Ideas to reduce and control herx reactions.
- Tips and clinical research from James Schaller, M.D.
- A detailed look at one method for utilizing antibiotics during a rife machine treatment campaign.
- Wide coverage of the Marshall Protocol, including an in-depth discussion of its mechanism of action in relation to Lyme disease pathology. Also, the author's personal experience with the Marshall Protocol over 3 years.
- An explanation of and new information about the Salt / Vitamin C protocol.
- Hot-off-the-press information on mangosteen fruit (not to be confused with mango) and its many benefits, including antibacterial, anti-inflammatory, and anti-cancer properties.
- New guidelines for combining all the therapies discussed in both of Rosner's books into a complete treatment plan. Brief and articulate for consideration by you and your doctor.
- Also includes updates on rife therapy, cutting-edge supplements, political challenges, an exclusive interview with Willy Burgdorfer, Ph.D. (discoverer of Lyme), and much more!

> "Bryan Rosner thinks big and this new book offers big solutions."
> **- James Schaller, M.D.**
>
> "Another ground-breaking Lyme Disease book."
> **- Jeff Mittelman, moderator of the Lyme-and-rife group**
>
> "Brilliant and thorough."
> **- Nenah Sylver, Ph.D.**

Do not miss this top Lyme disease resource. Discover new healing tools today! Bring this book to your doctor's appointment to help with forming a treatment plan.

Paperback book, 7 x 10", 367 pages, $35

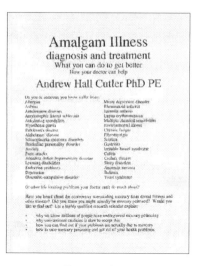

Book • $35

Amalgam Illness, Diagnosis and Treatment: What You Can Do to Get Better, How Your Doctor Can Help

By Andrew Cutler, PhD

This book was written by a chemical engineer who himself got mercury poisoning from his amalgam dental fillings. He found that there was no suitable educational material for either the patient or the physician. Knowing how much people can suffer from this condition, he wrote this book to help them get well. With a PhD in chemistry from Princeton University and extensive study in biochemistry and medicine, Andrew Cutler uses layman's terms to explain how people become mercury poisoned and what to do about it. The author's research shows that mercury poisoning can easily be cured at home with over-the-counter oral chelators – this book explains how.

In the book you will find practical guidance on how to tell if you really have chronic mercury poisoning or some other problem. Proper diagnostic procedures are provided so that sick people can decide what is wrong rather than trying random treatments. If mercury poisoning is your problem, the book tells you how to get the mercury out of your body, and how to feel good while you do that. The treatment section gives step-by-step directions to figure out exactly what mercury is doing to you and how to fix it.

"Dr. Cutler uses his background in chemistry to explain the safest approach to treat mercury poisoning. I am a physician and am personally using his protocol on myself."

- Melissa Myers, M.D.

Sections also explain how the scientific literature shows many people must be getting poisoned by their amalgam fillings, why such a regulatory blunder occurred, and how the debate between "mainstream" and "alternative" medicine makes it more difficult for you to get the medical help you need.

This down-to-earth book lets patients take care of themselves. It also lets doctors who are not familiar with chronic mercury intoxication treat it. The book is a practical guide to getting well. Sections from the book include:

- Why worry about mercury poisoning?
- What mercury does to you – symptoms, laboratory test irregularities, diagnostic checklist.
- How to treat mercury poisoning easily with oral chelators.
- Dealing with other metals including copper, arsenic, lead, cadmium.
- Dietary and supplement guidelines.
- Balancing hormones during the recovery process.
- How to feel good while you are chelating the metals out.
- How heavy metals cause infections to thrive in the body.
- Politics and mercury.

This is the world's most authoritative, accurate book on mercury poisoning.

Paperback book, 8.5 x 11", 226 pages, $35

Hair Test Interpretation: Finding Hidden Toxicities

By Andrew Cutler, PhD

Hair tests are worth doing because a surprising number of people diagnosed with incurable chronic health conditions actually turn out to have a heavy metal problem; quite often, mercury poisoning. Heavy metal problems can be corrected. Hair testing allows the underlying problem to be identified – and the chronic health condition often disappears with proper detoxification.

Hair Test Interpretation: Finding Hidden Toxicities is a practical book that explains how to interpret **Doctor's Data, Inc**. and **Great Plains Laboratory** hair tests. A step-by-step discussion is provided, with figures to illustrate the process and make it easy. The book gives examples using actual hair test results from real people.

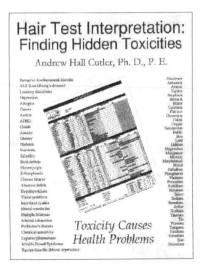

Hair Test Interpretation: Finding Hidden Toxicities
Andrew Hall Cutler, Ph. D., P. E.

Toxicity Causes Health Problems

Book • $35

One of the problems with hair testing is that both conventional and alternative health care providers do not know how to interpret these tests. Interpretation is not as simple as looking at the results and assuming that any mineral out of the reference range is a problem mineral.

Interpretation is complicated because heavy metal toxicity, especially mercury poisoning, interferes with mineral transport throughout the body. Ironically, if someone is mercury poisoned, hair test mercury is often low and other minerals may be elevated or take on unusual values. For example, mercury often causes retention of arsenic, antimony, tin, titanium, zirconium, and aluminum. An inexperienced health care provider may wrongfully assume that one of these other minerals is the culprit, when in reality mercury is the true toxicity.

"This new book of Andrew's is the definitive guide in the confusing world of heavy metal poisoning diagnosis and treatment. I'm a practicing physician, 20 years now, specializing in detoxification programs for treatment of resistant conditions. It was fairly difficult to diagnose these heavy metal conditions before I met Andrew Cutler and developed a close relationship with him while reading his books. In this book I found his usual painful attention to detail gave a solid framework for understanding the complexity of mercury toxicity as well as the less common exposures. You really couldn't ask for a better reference book on a subject most researchers and physicians are still fumbling in the dark about."
- Dr. Rick Marschall

So, as you can see, getting a hair test is only the first step. The second step is figuring out what the hair test means. Andrew Cutler, PhD, is a registered professional chemical engineer with years of experience in biochemical and healthcare research. This clear and concise book makes hair test interpretation easy, so that you know which toxicities are causing your health problems.

Paperback book, 8.5 x 11", 298 pages, $35

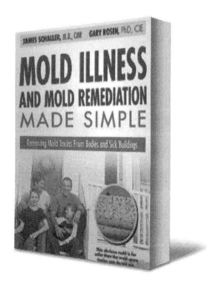

Book • $32.95

Mold Illness and Mold Remediation Made Simple: Removing Mold Toxins from Bodies and Sick Buildings

By James Schaller, M.D. and Gary Rosen, Ph.D.

Indoor mold toxins are much more dangerous and prevalent than most people realize. Visible mold in and around your house is far less dangerous than the mold you cannot see. Indoor mold toxicity, in addition to causing its own unique set of health problems and symptoms, also greatly contributes to the severity of most chronic illnesses.

In this book, a top physician and experienced contractor team up to help you quickly recover from indoor mold exposure. This book is easy to read with many color photographs and illustrations.

Dr. Schaller is a practicing physician in Florida who has written more than 15 books. He is one of the few physicians in the United States successfully treating mold toxin illness in children and adults.

Dr. Rosen is a biochemist with training under a Nobel Prize winning researcher at UCLA. He has written several books and is an expert in the mold remediation of homes. Dr. Rosen and his family are sensitive to mold toxins so he writes not only from professional experience, but also from personal experience.

Together, the two authors have certification in mold testing, mold remediation, and indoor environmental health. This book is one of the most complete on the subject, and includes discussion of the following topics:

- Potential mold problems encountered in new homes, schools, and jobs.
- Diagnosing mold illness.
- Mold as it relates to dryness and humidity.
- Mold toxins and cancer treatment.
- Mold toxins and relationships.
- Crawlspaces, basements, attics, home cleaning techniques, and vacuums.
- Training your eyes to discern indoor mold.
- Leptin and obesity.
- Appropriate/inappropriate air filters and cleaners.
- How to handle old, musty products, materials and books, and how to safely sterilize them.
- A description of various types of molds, images of them, and their relative toxicity.
- Blood testing and how to use it to find hidden health problems.
- The book is written in a friendly, casual tone that allows easy comprehension and information retention.

> "A concise, practical guide on dealing with mold toxins and their effects."
>
> **- Bryan Rosner**

Many people are affected by mold toxins. Are you? If you can find a smarter or clearer book on this subject, buy it!

Paperback book, 8.5 x 11", 140 pages, $32.95
Also available on our website as an eBook!

Treatment of Chronic Lyme Disease: 51 Case Reports and Essays In Their Regard

By Burton Waisbren Sr., MD, FACP, FIDSA

DON'T MISS THIS BOOK! A MUST-HAVE RESOURCE. What sets this Lyme disease book apart are the credentials of its author: he is not only a Fellow of the Infectious Diseases Society of America (IDSA), he is also one of its Founders! With 57+ years experience in medicine, Dr. Waisbren passionately argues for the validity of chronic Lyme disease and presents useful information about 51 cases of the disease which he has personally treated. His position is in stark contrast to that of the IDSA, which is a very powerful organization. **Quite possibly the most important book ever published on Lyme disease, as a result of the author's experience and credentials.**

Book • $24.95

Paperback book, 6x9", 169 pages, $24.95

Bartonella:
Diagnosis and Treatment

By James Schaller, M.D.

2 Book Set • $99.95

As an addition to his growing collection of informative books, Dr. James Schaller penned this excellent 2-part volume on Bartonella, a Lyme disease co-infection. The set is an ideal complementary resource to his Babesia textbook (next page).

Bartonella infections occur throughout the entire world, in cities, suburbs, and rural locations. It is found in fleas, dust mites, ticks, lice, flies, cat and dog saliva, and insect feces.

This 2-book set provides advanced treatment strategies as well as detailed diagnostic criteria, with dozens of full-color illustrations and photographs.

Both books in this 2-part set are included with your order.

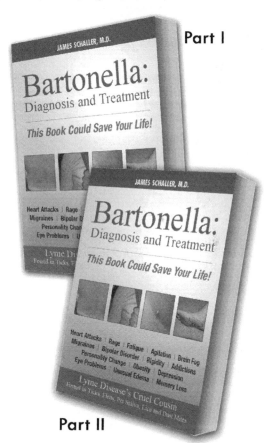

Part I

Part II

2 paperback books included, 7 x 10", 500 pages, $99.95

351

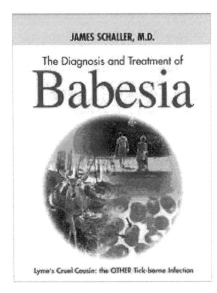

Book • $55

The Diagnosis and Treatment of Babesia: Lyme's Cruel Cousin – The Other Tick-Borne Infection

By James Schaller, M.D.

Do you or a loved one experience excess fatigue? Have you ever had unusually high fevers, chills, or sweats? You may have Babesia, a very common tick-borne infection. Babesia is often found with Lyme disease and, like all tick-borne infections, is rarely diagnosed and reported accurately.

The deer tick which carries Lyme disease and Babesia may be as small as a poppy seed and injects a painkiller, an antihistamine, and an anticoagulant to avoid detection. As a result, many people have Babesia and do not know it. Numerous forms of Babesia are carried by ticks. This book introduces patients and health care workers to the various species that infect humans and are not routinely tested for by sincere physicians.

Dr. Schaller, who practices medicine in Florida, first became interested in Babesia after one of his own children was infected with it. None of the elite pediatricians or child specialists could help. No one tested for Babesia or considered it a possible diagnosis. His child suffered from just two of these typical Babesia symptoms:

- Significant Fatigue
- Coughing
- Dizziness
- Trouble Thinking
- Fevers
- Memory Loss

- Chills
- Air Hunger
- Headache
- Sweats
- Unresponsiveness to Lyme Treatment

With 374 pages, this book is the most current and comprehensive book on Babesia in the English language. It reviews thousands of articles and presents the results of interviews with world experts on the subject. It offers you top information and broad treatment options, presented in a clear and simple manner. All treatments are explained thoroughly, including their possible side effects, drug interactions, various dosing strategies, pros/cons, and physician experiences.

"Once again Dr. Schaller has provided us with a much-needed and practical resource. This book gave me exactly what I was looking for."

- Thomas W., Patient

Finally, the book also addresses many other aspects of practical medical care often overlooked in this infection, such as treatment options for managing fatigue. Plainly stated, this book is a must-have for patients and health care providers who deal with Lyme disease and its co-infections. Dr. Schaller's many years in clinical practice give the book a practical angle that many other similar books lack. Don't miss this user-friendly resource!

Paperback book, 7 x 10", 374 pages, $55

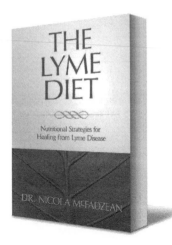

Book • $24.95

The Lyme Diet: Nutritional Strategies for Healing from Lyme Disease

By Nicola McFadzean, N.D.

We know about antibiotics and herbs. But what is the right diet for Lyme sufferers? Now you can read about the experience of Dr. Nicola McFadzean, N.D., in treating Lyme patients using proper diet.

The author is a Naturopathic Doctor and graduate of Bastyr University in Seattle, Washington. She is currently in private practice at her clinic, RestorMedicine, located in San Diego, California.

Nicola McFadzean, N.D.

This book covers numerous topics (not just diet-related):

- Reducing and controlling inflammation
- Maximizing immune function via dietary choices
- Restoring the gut & regaining healthy digestion
- Detoxification with food
- Hormone imbalances
- Biofilms
- Kefir vs. yogurt vs. probiotics
- Candida, liver support, and much more!

Paperback book, 6x9", 214 Pages, $24.95
Also available as an eBook on our website!

The Stealth Killer: Is Oral Spirochetosis the Missing Link in the Dental & Heart Disease Labyrinth? *By William D. Nordquist, BS, DMD, MS*

Can oral spirochete infections cause heart attacks? In today's cosmopolitan urban population, more than 51 percent of those with root canal–treated teeth probably have infection at the apex of their root. Dr. Nordquist, an oral surgeon practicing in Southern California, believes that any source of bacteria with resulting chronic infection (including periodontal disease) in the mouth may potentially lead to heart disease and other systemic diseases. With more than 40 illustrations and x-ray reproductions, this book takes you behind the scenes in Dr. Nordquist's research laboratory, and provides many tips on dealing with Lyme-related dental problems. A breakthrough book in dentistry & infectious disease!

Paperback Book • $25.95

Paperback book, 6x9", 161 pages, $25.95

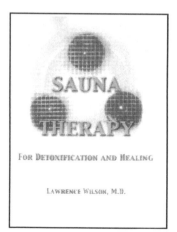

SAUNA THERAPY

FOR DETOXIFICATION AND HEALING

LAWRENCE WILSON, M.D.

Book • $22.95

Sauna Therapy for Detoxification and Healing

By Lawrence Wilson, MD

This book provides a thorough yet articulate education on sauna therapy. It includes construction plans for a low-cost electric light sauna. The book is well referenced with an extensive bibliography.

Sauna therapy, especially with an electric light sauna, is one of the most powerful, safe and cost-effective methods of natural healing. It is especially important today due to extensive exposure to toxic metals and chemicals.

Fifteen chapters cover sauna benefits, physiological effects, protocols, cautions, healing reactions, and many other aspects of sauna therapy.

Dr. Wilson is an instructor of Biochemistry, Hair Mineral Analysis, Sauna Therapy and Jurisprudence at various colleges and universities including Yamuni Institute of the Healing Arts (Maurice, LA), University of Natural Medicine (Santa Fe, NM), Natural Healers Academy (Morristown, NJ), and Westbrook University (West Virginia). His books are used as textbooks at East-West School of Herbology and Ohio College of Natural Health. Go to www.LymeBook.com for free book excerpts!.

Paperback book, 8.5 x 11", 167 pages, $22.95

Physicians' Desk Reference (PDR) Books (opposing page)

Most people have heard of *Physicians' Desk Reference* (PDR) books because, for over 60 years, physicians and researchers have turned to PDR for the latest word on prescription drugs.

You may not know that Thomson Healthcare, publisher of PDR, offers PDR reference books not only

THOMSON

"I relied heavily on the PDRs during the research phase of writing my books. Without them, my projects would have greatly suffered."

- Bryan Rosner

for drugs, but also for herbal and nutritional supplements. No available books come even close to the amount of information provided in these PDRs—*PDR for Herbal Medicines* weighs 5 lbs and has over 1300 pages, and *PDR for Nutritional Supplements* weighs over 3 lbs and has more than 800 pages.

We carry all three PDRs. Although PDR books are typically used by physicians, we feel that these resources are also essential for people interested in or recovering from chronic disease. For the supplements, herbs, and drugs included in the books, you will find the following information: Pharmacology, description and method of action, available trade names and brands, indications and usage, research summaries, dosage options, history of use, pharmacokinetics, and much more! Worth the money for years of faithful use.

PDR for Nutritional Supplements   *2nd Edition!*

This PDR focuses on the following types of supplements:

- Vitamins
- Minerals
- Amino acids
- Hormones
- Lipids
- Glyconutrients
- Probiotics
- Proteins
- Many more!

"In a part of the health field not known for its devotion to rigorous science, [this book] brings to the practitioner and the curious patient a wealth of hard facts."

- Roger Guillemin, M.D., Ph.D., Nobel Laureate in Physiology and Medicine

Book • $69.50

The book also suggests supplements that can help reduce prescription drug side effects, has full-color photographs of various popular commercial formulations (and contact information for the associated suppliers), and so much more! Become educated instead of guessing which supplements to take.

Hardcover book, 11 x 9.3", 800 pages, $69.50

PDR for Herbal Medicines   *4th Edition!*

PDR for Herbal Medicines is very well organized and presents information on hundreds of common and uncommon herbs and herbal preparations. Indications and usage are examined with regard to homeopathy, Indian and Chinese medicine, and unproven (yet popular) applications.

In an area of healthcare so unstudied and vulnerable to hearsay and hype, this scientifically referenced book allows you to find out the real story behind the herbs lining the walls of your local health food store.

Use this reference before spending money on herbal products!

Book • $69.50

Hardcover book, 11 x 9.3", 1300 pages, $69.50

PDR for Prescription Drugs   *Current Year's Edition!*

With more than 3,000 pages, this is the most comprehensive and respected book in the world on over 4,000 drugs. Drugs are indexed by both brand and generic name (in the same convenient index) and also by manufacturer and product category. This PDR provides usage information and warnings, drug interactions, plus a detailed, full-color directory with descriptions and cross references for the drugs. A new format allows dramatically improved readability and easier access to the information you need now.

Book • $99.50

Hardcover book, 12.5 x 9.5", 3533 pages, $99.50

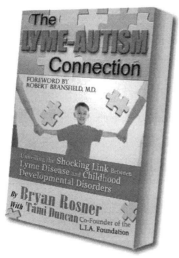

Book • $25.95

The Lyme-Autism Connection: Unveiling the Shocking Link Between Lyme Disease and Childhood Developmental Disorders
By Bryan Rosner & Tami Duncan

Did you know that Lyme disease may contribute to the onset of autism?

This book is an investigative report written by Bryan Rosner and Tami Duncan. Duncan is the co-founder of the *Lyme Induced Autism (LIA) Foundation*, and her son has an autism diagnosis.

Tami Duncan, Co-Founder of the Lyme Induced Autism (LIA) Foundation

Awareness of the Lyme-autism connection is spreading rapidly, among both parents and practitioners. *Medical Hypothesis*, a scientific, peer-reviewed journal published by Elsevier, recently released an influential study entitled *The Association Between Tick-Borne Infections, Lyme Borreliosis and Autism Spectrum Disorders*. Here is an excerpt from the study:

> "Chronic infectious diseases, including tick-borne infections such as Borrelia burgdorferi, may have direct effects, promote other infections, and create a weakened, sensitized and immunologically vulnerable state during fetal development and infancy, leading to increased vulnerability for developing autism spectrum disorders. An association between Lyme disease and other tick-borne infections and autistic symptoms has been noted by numerous clinicians and parents."

—**Medical Hypothesis Journal.**
Article Authors: Robert C. Bransfield, M.D., Jeffrey S. Wulfman, M.D., William T. Harvey, M.D., Anju I. Usman, M.D.

Nationwide, 1 out of 150 children are diagnosed with Autism Spectrum Disorder (ASD), and the LIA Foundation has discovered that many of these children test positive for Lyme disease/Borrelia related complex—yet most children in this scenario never receive appropriate medical attention. This book answers many difficult questions: How can infants contract Lyme disease if autism begins before birth, precluding the opportunity for a tick bite? Is there a statistical correlation between the incidences of Lyme disease and autism worldwide? Do autistic children respond to Lyme disease treatment? What does the medical community say about this connection? Do the mothers of affected children exhibit symptoms? **Find out in this book.**

Paperback book, 6x9", 287 pages, $25.95

Dietrich Klinghardt, M.D., Ph.D.
"Fundamental Teachings"
5-DVD Set

Includes Disc Exclusively For Lyme Disease!

Dietrich Klinghardt, M.D., Ph.D. is a legendary healer known for discovering and refining many of the cutting-edge treatment protocols used for a variety of chronic health problems including Lyme disease, autism and mercury poisoning.

Now you can find out all about this doctor's treatment methods from the privacy of your own home! This 5-DVD set includes the following DVDs:

- **DISC 1**: The Five Levels of Healing and the Seven Factors

- **DISC 2**: Autonomic Response Testing and Demonstration

- **DISC 3**: Heavy Metal Toxicity and Neurotoxin Elimination / Electrosmog

- **DISC 4**: Lyme disease and Chronic Illness

- **DISC 5**: Psycho-Emotional Issues in Chronic Illness & Addressing Underlying Causes

5-DVD Set • $125

Dr. Dietrich Klinghardt is one of the most important contributors to modern integrative treatment for Lyme disease and related medical conditions. This comprehensive DVD set is a must-have addition to your educational library.

5-DVD Set, $125

Our catalog has space limitations, but our website does not! Visit www.LymeBook.com to see even more exciting products.

Don't Miss These New Books & DVDs, Available Online:
- Babesia Update 2009, by James Schaller, M.D.
- Marshall Protocol 5-DVD Set
- Cure Unknown, by Pamela Weintraub
- The Experts of Lyme Disease, by Sue Vogan
- The Lyme Disease Solution, by Ken Singleton, M.D.
- **Lots of Free Chapters and Excerpts Online!**

Don't use the internet? No problem, just call (530) 573-0190.

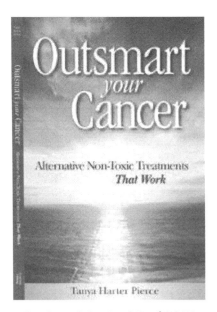

Book and Audio CD • $24.50

**Outsmart Your Cancer:
Alternative Non-Toxic Treatments
That Work   By Tanya Harter Pierce**

Why BLUDGEON cancer to death with common conventional treatments that can be toxic and harmful to your entire body?

When you OUTSMART your cancer, only the cancer cells die — NOT your healthy cells! *OUTSMART YOUR CANCER: Alternative Non-Toxic Treatments That Work* is an easy guide to successful non-toxic treatments for cancer that you can obtain right now! In it, you will read real-life stories of people who have completely recovered from their advanced or late-stage lung cancer, breast cancer, prostate cancer, kidney cancer, brain cancer, childhood leukemia, and other types of cancer using effective non-toxic approaches.

Plus, *OUTSMART YOUR CANCER* is one of the few books in print today that gives a complete description of the amazing formula called "Protocel," which has produced incredible cancer recoveries over the past 20 years. **A supporting audio CD is included with this book**. Pricing = $19.95 book + $5.00 CD.

Paperback book, 6 x 9", 437 pages, with audio CD, $24.95

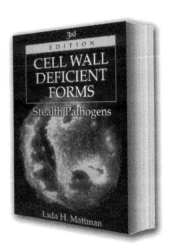

Hardcover Book • $169.95

Cell Wall Deficient Forms: Stealth Pathogens

By Lida Mattman, Ph.D.

This is one of the most influential infectious disease textbook of the century. Dr. Mattman, who earned a Ph.D. in immunology from Yale University, describes her discovery that a certain type of pathogen lacking a cell wall is the root cause of many of today's "incurable" and mysterious chronic diseases. Dr. Mattman's research is the foundation of our current understanding of Lyme disease, and her work led to many of the Lyme protocols used today (such as the Marshall Protocol, as well as modern LLMD antibiotic treatment strategy). Color illustrations and meticulously referenced breakthrough principles cover the pages of this book. A must have for all serious students of chronic, elusive infectious disease.

Hardcover book, 7.5 x 10.5", 416 pages, $169.95

318

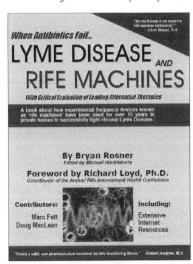

Book • $35

When Antibiotics Fail: Lyme Disease And Rife Machines, With Critical Evaluation Of Leading Alternative Therapies

By Bryan Rosner
Foreword by Richard Loyd, Ph.D.

There are enough books and websites about what Lyme disease is and which ticks carry it. But there is very little useful information for people who actually have a case of Lyme disease that is not responding to conventional antibiotic treatment. Lyme disease sufferers need to know their options, not how to identify a tick.

This book describes how experimental electromagnetic frequency devices known as rife machines have been used for over 15 years in private homes to fight Lyme disease. Also included are evaluations of more than 25 conventional and alternative Lyme disease therapies, including:

- Homeopathy
- IV and oral antibiotics
- Mercury detox.
- Hyperthermia / saunas
- Ozone and oxygen
- Samento®
- Colloidal Silver
- Bacterial die-off detox.

- Colostrum
- Magnesium supplementation
- Hyperbaric oxygen chamber (HBOC)
- ICHT Italian treatment
- Non-pharmaceutical antibiotics
- Exercise, diet and candida protocols
- Cyst-targeting antibiotics
- The Marshall Protocol®

Many Lyme disease sufferers have heard of rife machines, some have used them. But until now, there has not been a concise and organized source to explain how and why they have been used by Lyme patients. In fact, this is the first book ever published on this important topic.

The Foreword for the book is by Richard Loyd, Ph.D., coordinator of the annual Rife International Health Conference. The book takes a practical, down-to-earth approach which allows you to learn about*:

> "This book provides life-saving insights for Lyme disease patients."
>
> **- Richard Loyd, Ph.D.**

- Antibiotic treatment problems and shortcomings—why some people choose to use rife machines after other therapies fail.
- Hypothetical treatment schedules and sessions, based on the author's experience.
- The experimental machines with the longest track record: High Power Magnetic Pulser, EMEM Machine, Coil Machine, and AC Contact Machine.
- Explanation of the "herx reaction" and why it may indicate progress.
- The intriguing story that led to the use of rife machines to fight Lyme disease 20 years ago.
- Antibiotic categories and classifications, with pros and cons of each type of drug.
- Visit our website to read FREE EXCERPTS from the book!

*****Disclaimer:** Your treatment decisions must be made under the care of a licensed physician. Rife machines are not FDA approved and the FDA has not reviewed or approved of these books. The author is a layperson, not a doctor, and much of the content of these books is a statement of opinion based on the author's personal experience and research.*

Paperback book, 8.5 x 11", 203 pages, $35

**Under Our Skin:
Lyme Disease Documentary
Film**

A gripping tale of microbes, medicine & money, UNDER OUR SKIN exposes the hidden story of Lyme disease, one of the most serious and controversial epidemics of our time. Each year, thousands go undiagnosed or misdiagnosed, often told that their symptoms are all in their head.

DVD • $34.95

Following the stories of patients and physicians fighting for their lives and livelihoods, the film brings into focus a haunting picture of the health care system and a medical establishment all too willing to put profits ahead of patients.

Bonus Features: 32-page discussion guidebook, one hour of bonus footage, director's commentary, and much more! **FOR HOME USE ONLY**

DVD with bonus features, 104 minutes, $34.95 *MUST SEE!*

Ordering is Easy! Phone: **Toll Free (866) 476-7637**
Online: **www.LymeBook.com**

Detailed product information and secure online ordering is available on our website. Bulk orders to bookstores, health food stores, or Lyme disease support groups – call us for wholesale terms.

Do you have a book inside you? Submit your book proposal online at: www.lymebook.com/submit-book-proposal.

Join Lyme Community Forums at: www.lymecommunity.com.

Get paid to help us place our books in your local health food store. Learn more: www.lymebook.com/local-store-offer.

DISCLAIMER

This disclaimer is in reference to all books, DVDs, websites, flyers, and catalogs published by Bryan Rosner, DBA BioMed Publishing Group.

Our materials are for informational and educational purposes only. They are not intended to prevent, diagnose, treat, or cure disease. Some of the treatments described are not FDA-Approved. Bryan Rosner is a layperson, not a medical professional, and he is not qualified to dispense medical advice.

These books and DVDs are not intended to substitute for professional medical care. Do not postpone receiving care from a licensed physician. Please read our full disclaimer online at: www.lymebook.com/homepage-disclaimer.pdf.

INDEX

M

N

O

P

Z

ABOUT THE AUTHOR

Dr. Nicola McFadzean is the founder and Medical Director of Restor-Medicine, an integrative medical center based in San Diego, CA. Having done her naturopathic training and completed her Bachelor of Health Sciences in Australia, she moved to the United States and obtained her Doctorate of Naturopathic Medicine from Bastyr University, starting a private practice in Southern California soon thereafter.

Dr. Nicola is a Lyme-literate Naturopathic Physician, combining conventional and integrative approaches to treating Lyme and other tick-borne illness. She is a member of the International Lyme and Associated Diseases Society (ILADS) and has completed the ILADS Physician Training Program under the mentorship of Steven Harris, MD.

Dr. McFadzean is the author of *The Lyme Diet: Nutritional Strategies for Healing From Lyme Disease* and *Lyme Disease in Australia: Fundamentals of an Emerging Epidemic,* and is a chapter contributor to Connie Strasheim's book *Insights into Lyme Disease Treatment: 13 Lyme-literate Practitioners Share Their Healing Strategies.*

She conducts Lyme disease clinics in Australia twice a year, helping Lyme-sufferers navigate the testing and treatment options for tick-borne illness; and is the Medical Advisor to the Lyme Disease Association of Australia.

Consultations with Dr. Nicola are scheduled through RestorMedicine's home office in San Diego. RestorMedicine can be contacted via phone at 1 (619) 546 4065 or by email – **info@restormedicine.com.** Patients can also schedule their own appointments online by going to **www.restormedicine.com** and following the "schedule a consultation" link. Dr. Nicola works with patients both throughout the United States and internationally via telephone or Skype.

15166466R00193

Made in the USA
Charleston, SC
20 October 2012